C 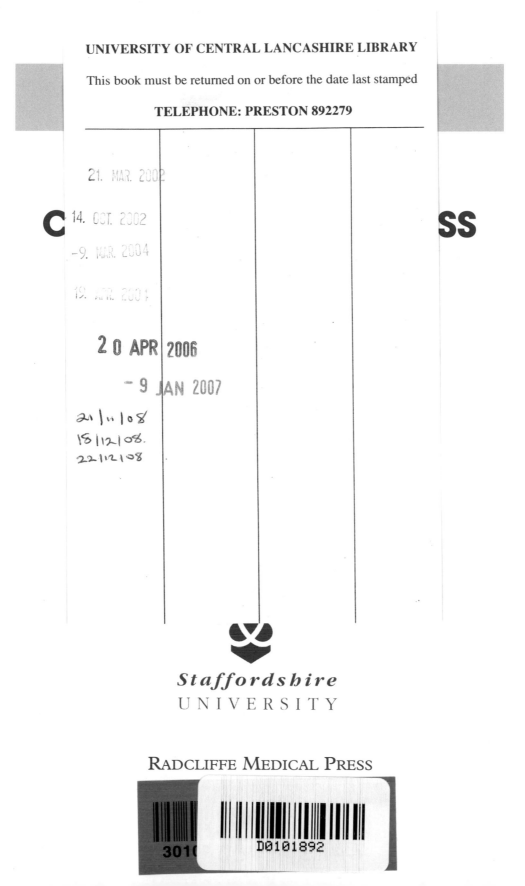 SS

Staffordshire
UNIVERSITY

RADCLIFFE MEDICAL PRESS

©2001 Anne Weston, Ruth Chambers and Elizabeth Boath
Illustrations ©2001 Martin Davies

Radcliffe Medical Press Ltd
18 Marcham Road, Abingdon, Oxon OX14 1AA

British Library Cataloguing in Publication Data

A catalogue record for this book is available from the British Library.

ISBN 1 85775 449 2

Typeset by Advance Typesetting Ltd, Oxon
Printed and bound by TJ International Ltd, Padstow, Cornwall

► CONTENTS

Stage 2: Undertaking a library search   39

Stage 3: Frame your own question and search for the evidence   57

Stage 4: Appraise the evidence   63

Stage 5: Apply the evidence   103

► ABOUT THE AUTHORS

Anne Weston has been a midwife since 1982 and in midwifery education since 1987. Currently she is Principal Lecturer for Midwifery at the School of Health, Staffordshire University. Her interest in clinical effectiveness and clinical governance relating to midwifery practice grew out of participating in one of Ruth's clinical effectiveness workshops. Anne is committed to promoting evidence-based midwifery practice and practice development.

Ruth Chambers has been a general practitioner for 22 years. She is currently Professor of Primary Care Development at the Centre for Health Policy and Practice, Staffordshire University. Her interest in clinical effectiveness and clinical audit grew during her three-year spell as Chairman of Staffordshire Medical Audit Advisory Group until 1996.

Ruth has run several series of clinical effectiveness and clinical governance workshops, teaching a mix of primary and community care health professionals clinical effectiveness skills in easy steps and an understanding of clinical governance. The experiences of those workshops have informed this book.

Elizabeth Boath is the Head of the Centre for Health Policy and Practice at the School of Health, Staffordshire University. Her interest in clinical effectiveness grew from her time as a primary and community care research facilitator, during which she facilitated and taught on the series of clinical effectiveness workshops used to develop this book.

► ACKNOWLEDGEMENTS

The workshops and composition of this book were developed with a grant from the regional Evidence-supported Medicine Union (EMU) and funding from the Staffordshire and Shropshire Non-Medical Education Consortium, to improve evidence-based care in the West Midlands.

North Staffordshire Medical Audit Advisory Group were joint organisers of the clinical effectiveness workshop series and North Staffordshire Combined Healthcare NHS Trust was co-host of many of the clinical governance workshops.

The book is based upon the experiences from running two series of four workshops, *Clinical Effectiveness Made Easy*, for primary and community care practitioners and 20 workshops about *Clinical Governance*. We are grateful to the participants of the workshops for contributing so many ideas and being such an enthusiastic bunch of health professionals. Irene Fenton and David Rogers, medical librarians, provided the inspiration and clear advice about undertaking literature searches and other sources of evidence.

We are grateful to Nicky Macleod for her contribution about the meaning of cost-effectiveness, and Dr Gill Wakley who helped to devise and facilitate the clinical governance workshops.

Anne Weston
Ruth Chambers
Elizabeth Boath
April 2001

'Many popular beliefs are either logically wrong or are not supported by evidence … There is no confusion more dangerous than the plausible.'

Normand C (1998) Ten popular health economic fallacies. *Public Health Medicine.* **20**(2): 129–32.

Clinical effectiveness and clinical governance are about knowing what you should be doing and being able to put that knowledge into practice

Overall aim of the programme

To increase awareness of, and skills in, the adoption of an evidence-based approach to the practice and delivery of midwifery care.

Objectives of this book

This programme is for midwives to learn how to:

▶ ask the right question – it must be important to you and your colleagues
▶ look for the evidence and do a library search
▶ receive and incorporate constructive criticism from colleagues about their developing questions and search for evidence
▶ select the best evidence – what to do where none exists
▶ evaluate and interpret the evidence, such as read and extract information from a report
▶ apply the evidence as appropriate in practice

- ▸ act on the evidence to improve the practice of clinical effectiveness
- ▸ promote a culture of clinical governance.

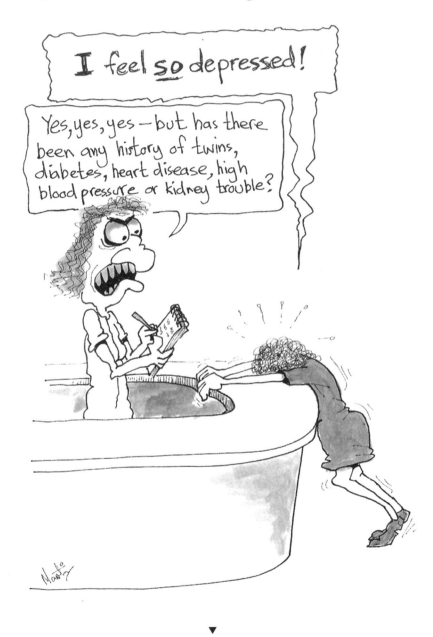

▼

Do you need to update your style of practice?

Self-assessment of where you are now with clinical effectiveness and clinical governance

Before you start working through the clinical effectiveness and clinical governance programme, assess your baseline knowledge and attitudes. Please circle as many answers as apply, or fill in the information requested.

1 How confident do you feel that you are capable of practising clinical effectiveness to be able to:

ask a relevant question?	*Very*	*Somewhat*	*Not at all*
undertake a search of the literature?	*Very*	*Somewhat*	*Not at all*
find readily available evidence?	*Very*	*Somewhat*	*Not at all*
weigh up available evidence?	*Very*	*Somewhat*	*Not at all*
decide if changes in practice are warranted?	*Very*	*Somewhat*	*Not at all*
make changes in practice as appropriate?	*Very*	*Somewhat*	*Not at all*

2 Have you ever searched the literature yourself for an answer to a question? *Yes / No*

If '*Yes*':

▶ which database(s) have you used?
>   *CINAHL   Medline   Cochrane   Internet   Other (what?)*

▶ where did you search the literature?
>   *Library   At work   At home   Other (where?)*

▶ did you have any help in searching the literature?
>   *None   Librarian   Friend/family   Work colleague   Other (who?)*

3 Have you ever asked someone else to search the literature for you? *Yes / No*

If '*Yes*':

▶ who did the search for you?

▶ why didn't you do the search yourself?
>   *Lack of time   Lack of skill   Lack of access   Other reason*
>   *to databases*

4 Can you complete the following list from your own knowledge, describing the features of different types or levels of evidence in decreasing order of robustness from very strong evidence to none at all?

Type	Features
I	Strong evidence from at least one systematic review of multiple, well-designed, randomised controlled trials
II	
III	
IV	
V	
VI	No evidence at all

5 If you have previously searched for the evidence to answer a question you had posed, what did you do with the result of your search? (Circle all that apply.)

▶ *Discussed it with colleagues at work*

▶ *Discussed it with friends or family*

▶ *Made change(s) to an aspect of work*

▶ *Decided against making any change(s) to any aspect of work*

▶ *Other outcome – what?*

6 To what extent is evidence-based healthcare central to your own practice? (Circle all that apply.)

▶ *I have no idea whether my everyday practice is evidence-based most of the time*

▶ *I assume that my everyday practice is evidence-based whenever possible, but I've no evidence for that assumption*

▶ *I ensure that my everyday practice is evidence-based by regularly comparing my practice against published standards of best practice and making appropriate changes*

7 How many of these principles of good practice in clinical governance do you generally include as part of your quality improvement work? (Circle all that apply.)

▶ *I actively promote or participate in multidisciplinary working*

▶ *I address national, local, organisational or professional priorities in my work*

▶ *I try to achieve partnership working, e.g. between agencies, between management/midwives*

▶ *I incorporate input from patients in my work (e.g. users, carers, the public), in training, planning, monitoring or delivery of healthcare*

▶ *I look for potential to achieve health gains in the way I organise my work*

▶ *My everyday work is based on evidence-based practice, policy or management*

▶ *I can demonstrate the standards of care or services that I or my team achieve.*

Find out how to practise clinical effectiveness – don't shut your eyes to the changes going on around you.

What are clinical effectiveness and evidence-based healthcare?

Clinical effectiveness is 'the extent to which specific clinical interventions, when deployed in the field for a particular patient or population, do what they are intended to do – i.e. maintain and improve health and secure the greatest possible health gain from the available resources. To be reasonably certain that an intervention has produced health benefits, it needs to be shown to be capable of producing worthwhile benefit (efficacy and cost-effectiveness) and that it has produced that benefit in practice'.[1]

Evidence-based healthcare 'takes place when decisions that affect the care of patients are taken with due weight accorded to all valid, relevant information'.[2]

Evidence-based medicine (EBM) is the 'conscientious, explicit, and judicious use of current best evidence in making decisions about the care of individual patients. The practice of evidence-based medicine means integrating individual clinical expertise with the best available external clinical evidence from systematic research'.[3]

A problem-solving approach based upon good evidence can also be applied to non-clinical decision making, such as most areas of management and resource allocation, as well as to clinical situations.

The three components of best possible clinical decision making[4,5] are *clinical expertise, patient preferences* and *clinical research evidence*. Clinical expertise and patient preferences may override the research evidence in some situations and for some patients. For example, patients may opt for less invasive treatment, or may choose not to have alpha foetoprotein screening.

Clinical audit remains an important tool for determining whether actual performance compares with evidence-based standards and, if not, what changes are needed to improve performance. Clinical audit is 'the systematic and critical analysis of the quality of clinical care, including the procedures used for diagnosis, treatment and care, the associated use of resources and the resulting outcome and quality of life for the patient'.[1] In other words, clinical audit helps you to reach a standard of clinical work as near to best practice as possible.

The process of achieving evidence-based practice can be divided into four sections:

1 the composition of a good question

2 a search of the literature to find the 'best' evidence available

3 an evaluation of what seems to be the most appropriate and relevant literature

4 the application of the evidence or findings.

What is the evidence for evidence-based healthcare?

There is growing evidence for the implementation of evidence-based healthcare.[6] Promoting Action on Clinical Effectiveness (PACE), a King's Fund programme, is developing evidence-based practice as a routine way of working for health services. An interim report[6] has described the successful outcomes when clinical effectiveness is linked to local needs and priorities so long as clinicians, managers, policy makers and patients are all involved in the process.

Practising in an evidence-based way:

▶ will promote your job satisfaction and feeling of being in control over your work
▶ can be used to justify maintaining or increasing budget allocations to particular areas of work
▶ will enhance your capability to do what's best for the patient.[7]

Why midwives need information

Midwives need to be well informed to be able to advise and inform patients appropriately. Patients who access the Internet and other electronic databases are starting to use that information to challenge midwives' decisions about their care.

Midwives will come under more pressure to respond to patients who have easy access to detailed information obtained from various sources, some of which will be inaccurate and misleading. The movement to women-centred care has been generally welcomed, but may be threatening for midwives who are insufficiently prepared to talk to well-informed patients, because they are unsure of their own knowledge base, are time pressured, or do not understand how to assess what is the best evidence.

Midwives will need to develop skills in finding and judging midwifery medical information, and communicating such information to patients appropriately. Midwives may lay themselves open to complaints or legal procedures if they fail to adopt best practice through ignorance of the available evidence. Midwives need good communication skills as well as reliable information when advising patients.

In the future, patients will be increasingly encouraged to seek out information from the Internet themselves. Midwives can help patients by indicating which electronic sources are most likely to be appropriate and reliable.

Ultimately, reliable and accurate information, good communication skills and patient empowerment are all features of a good quality maternity service and a positive culture of clinical governance. Midwives and managers need good information when assessing the health needs of their patient population, commissioning healthcare services, and striving to reduce inequalities between different sub-groups of their population or to reduce variations in performance between different practitioners.

Quality of care may be compromised ...

... without clinical effectiveness.

Are midwives ready for evidence-based healthcare?

Recent surveys of health professionals' perceptions of evidence-based medicine[7,8] found that they knew little about extracting information from journals, reviewing publications and databases, and that few who were knowledgeable used these sources of information. Twenty per cent had access to bibliographic databases in their surgeries and 17% had access to the worldwide web.[7] But the majority of health professionals welcomed evidence-based medicine and agreed that it improves patient care.[7] Health professionals have been found to be more aware of publications that summarise evidence,[9] such as *Bandolier* and *Effective Health Care Bulletins*, rather than electronic databases. The researchers[7] concluded that the way forward in encouraging primary care clinicians to adopt evidence-based healthcare lay in promoting and improving access to summaries of evidence, and encouraging those primary care clinicians who are skilled in accessing and interpreting evidence to develop local evidence-based guidelines and advice.

One study[8] concluded that what was needed was a culture whereby health professionals posed 'regular questions about the validity of patient care' and developed 'skills both in defining useful questions and finding the answers'.

Adverse comments about evidence-based practice include fear of the imposition of too rigid a healthcare culture, the loss of an overriding duty to provide compassionate and sensitive care[10] and that wholesale evidence-based practice is unrealistic because it is not affordable.[11] Some people mistrust the research–evidence base component of evidence-based practice because of the unreliability of some of the published literature; study biases are not always sufficiently recognised or acknowledged and, in occasional cases, have been discredited by sensational scandals involving researchers falsifying data.[12]

A needs assessment of multidisciplinary clinical staff working in acute trusts[13] discovered significant unease about the conversion from a clinical audit to a clinical effectiveness culture, let alone the further evolution to a clinical governance culture. Several practical difficulties constraining the uptake of evidence-based healthcare were a recurring theme: poor access to information and electronic databases, lack of understanding about the definition and advantages of evidence-based practices, and the widespread need for staff training in critical appraisal skills.

The Get Research Into Practice (GRIP) project in the West Midlands[14] has described many ways to accelerate the adoption of evidence-based practice and associated skills. The Aggressive Research Intelligence Facility (ARIF), which is a collaboration between public health, epidemiology, general practice and health service management centres, exists to advance the use of evidence in the provision of healthcare in the West Midlands region. ARIF's regular reports describe the reviews and appraisals of the evidence the unit has provided in response to questions posed mainly by purchasers. The answers can be duplicated when others request the same information.

Learning by portfolio

Portfolio-based learning has been promoted since the early 1990s as a style of education that allows individuals to progress at their own pace. People can adopt education relevant to their needs, and composing a portfolio allows plenty of opportunities for reflection. Portfolio-based learning is not an easy option[15] compared to relatively passive types of learning such as listening to lectures. It takes a great deal of effort to complete a successful portfolio built on your past experiences and to progress through the stages of gathering and processing new information, critical reflection, interpretation and application. But it is worth it. The satisfaction that comes from completing a portfolio is as much about being in control of your own education as about acquiring new knowledge, attitudes and/or skills.[16,17]

Achievement of your professional registration requirements, set out by the UKCC (United Kingdom Central Council for Nursing, Midwifery and Health Visiting) in PREP (Post Registration Education and Practice) is demonstrated through the development of a professional portfolio.[18] The main aim of PREP is to improve standards of care thus mirroring the focus of clinical effectiveness and clinical governance. You can combine meeting the requirements of PREP with practising clinical effectiveness and demonstrate the achievement of both through reflective writing in your portfolio.

Another advantage of composing a portfolio is that on-the-job learning is relevant to your work and life, and this is likely to retain your interest. At the end of the project you will have discovered that you have further educational and developmental needs. You will then have to decide whether or not you have taken learning about this topic, as to how to practise clinical effectiveness, as far as your resources permit (time, cost and effort).

So, using a portfolio-based approach to acquire the basic ability to practise clinical effectiveness, you should aim in your work programme to:

▶ identify the learning task(s), e.g. what capability you need to be able to practise clinical effectiveness and clinical governance
▶ set learning goals, e.g. learn to frame a question; search for, interpret and apply the evidence
▶ identify ways of achieving your goals by, for example, working through this book, peer group discussion, visiting colleagues, undertaking a (supervised) library search, exploring the Internet, reading more widely, making changes at work. Use this information to compose your personal development plan
▶ identify learning resources, e.g. the books and electronic databases in the library, the Internet, books, journals, video tuition tapes, local courses, correspondence from specialists
▶ monitor how well the learning is going, e.g. reflect on the development of your knowledge and skills, seek a colleague's view of your work. Work with others in your practice or at the trust, to feed your learning needs into the workplace development plan
▶ list your achievements, e.g. run through a cycle of clinical effectiveness
▶ use what you have learned, e.g. make change(s) at work as a result of obtaining evidence or new information as part of clinical governance.

Some people prefer to work alone, whilst others find that having a mentor to help build the portfolio is useful. A mentor can help to assess learning needs, develop a study plan, support and challenge the work done, identify further learning gaps, and generally help the person being mentored to stay on course. To some extent the way that this clinical effectiveness learning programme is set out obviates the need for a mentor, but if you think a mentor might facilitate your work, consider asking the supervisor of midwives to act as a mentor; or maybe a colleague could work alongside you sharing the course too, as a 'co-mentor' or 'buddy'.[15]

Clinical effectiveness requires real commitment.

Electronic databases

Although the databases listed below may not all seem immediately relevant to midwives, they actually are, as midwives need to be familiar with the full range of medical conditions.

The Internet

The Internet is the largest computer network in the world to which almost any type of computer can link. Most academic institutions are connected to the Joint Academic Network (JANET) and its Internet service (JIPS); staff and students can then access the Internet free on campus, or can dial up from home via a modem for the cost of a local phone call. Once an NHS-wide network is established there is the potential for NHS staff to have similar access to the Internet.

Information can be extracted from the Internet or exchanged via the worldwide web (www) by electronic mail, telnet, newsgroups, network news, file transfer protocol and gopher-space (a system of interlinked menus which allows access to many Internet resources). The worldwide web is a system for providing access to a network of interlinked documents and information services across the Internet. Documents can be stored on the web as text, images, sound or video. The language that the web clients and servers use to communicate with each other is called 'hypertext transfer protocol' (http).

To use the worldwide web you need software called a *browser* (or *client*) to view www documents, such as *Netscape*. If you want to read more about searching the Internet, further details are given in the reference section at the back of this book.[19]

Various companies such as CompuServe and Microsoft Network offer online services. CompuServe provides access to shopping services, technical support, world news, and so on. CompuServe also links into the wider world of the Internet.

Cochrane Library

http://www.cochrane.co.uk. 'This [the Cochrane Library] is the single best source of reliable evidence about the effects of healthcare'.[20] The Cochrane library includes:

- ▶ The Cochrane Database of Systematic Reviews (CDSR). These are structured, systematic reviews of controlled trials. Evidence is included or excluded according to explicit quality criteria. A meta-analysis is undertaken by combining data from different studies to increase the *power* of the findings.
- ▶ The Database of Abstracts of Reviews of Effectiveness (DARE). This is a database of research reviews of the effectiveness of healthcare interventions and the management and organisation of health services. The reviews are critically appraised by reviewers at the NHS Centre for Reviews and Dissemination at the University of York.
- ▶ The Cochrane Controlled Trials Register (CCTR). This bibliography of controlled trials has been compiled by hand searches through the world's literature. The Register includes reports from conference proceedings.
- ▶ Only the Cochrane Database of Systematic Reviews (CDSR) is available on the Internet. The other titles from the Cochrane Library are currently available through Update Software's CD-ROM. Negotiations are currently underway to bring the other Cochrane Library titles to the Internet. So, hopefully, the full library will be available soon. Details of the Cochrane Library and CDSR are available online at http://www.update-software.com/cochrane/cochrane-frame.html.

Medline

Medline is freely available on the Internet. Medline is available on CD-ROM or online via a PC (you will need a modem). It is produced by the National Library of Medicine in the United States.

Medline contains over 10 million citations dating from 1966 to the present, drawn from bibliographic citations and author abstracts from more than 4000 biomedical journals published in the United States and 70 other countries. Abstracts are available for about 70% of the entries. It covers the whole field of medicine, dentistry, veterinary medicine, medical psychology, nursing/midwifery, the healthcare system, and the pre-clinical sciences. Coverage is worldwide, but most records are from English-language sources or have English abstracts. It is available free through HealthGate at http://www.healthgate.com/. Medline is also available on CD-ROM through Silver Platter and Ovid Technologies, though beware as there are differences in search terms between the two.

EMBASE

The Excerpta Medica database (EMBASE) is one of the leading databases of biomedical literature that offers 13 comprehensive databases that are searched separately. These are: anaesthesiology; cardiology; drugs & pharmacology; gastroenterology; immunology & AIDS; nephrology; neurosciences; obstetrics & gynaecology; pathology; pediatrics; psychiatry; radiology & nuclear medicine; and rehabilitation. The references found in each database are indexed and abstracted from over 3500 biomedical journals beginning in 1988, but for drugs and pharmacology from 1990. It is updated monthly. Although over 40% of entries are drug related, EMBASE also covers areas such as health policy, drug and alcohol dependence, psychiatry, forensic science and pollution control. It is more up to date than Medline and offers worldwide coverage with a European focus.

Searching and browsing the titles of the references that your search finds is free. However, you need to pay to display the full reference (journal citation, author and abstract when available). EMBASE* is not a full text database, but you can order full text copies from this database for a fee. It is available at http://www.bids.ac.uk/embase.html.

CINAHL

The Cumulative Index to Nursing and Allied Health Literature (CINAHL) database, compiled by CINAHL Information Systems in the USA, is a comprehensive database of more than 1200 English language journals from 1982 to the present. Updated monthly, CINAHL covers all aspects of nursing and allied health disciplines, such as health education, occupational therapy, physical therapy, emergency services, and social services and healthcare. Selected journals are also indexed in the areas of consumer health, biomedicine, and health sciences librarianship. The database also provides access to healthcare books, nursing dissertations, selected conference proceedings, standards of professional practice, educational software and audio-visual materials in nursing. CINAHL has more than 7000 records with full text and 1200 records with images. Online abstracts are available for more than 800 of these journals. Approximately 70% of CINAHL headings also appear in Medline. CINAHL supplements these headings with 2000+ terms designed specifically for nursing and allied health. For more information, see the following website: http://www.cinahl.com. Email: support@cinahl.com.

Several studies have compared Medline and CINAHL. These revealed that while Medline assigns more index terms to each article, CINAHL uses index terms that are more focused on nursing and therapy topics.[21] Another study revealed that CINAHL was preferred by nursing students as it gave a higher number of relevant articles, while another study found that both databases were relevant for professions allied to medicine (PAMs).[22,23] The authors concluded that, in order to ensure that the search is comprehensive, *both* Medline and CINAHL should be used.

Subject-specific bibliographic databases[24,25]

Over 2 000 000 articles are published each year in over 20 000 medical and related journals. Thus, although electronic databases provide access to references from a large number of journals, no database provides access to all journals. So, if you search only one or two databases, you might miss a relevant article. In addition to searching the main databases, it is also worthwhile searching any specialist databases relevant to your area of interest. Some of these databases are outlined in alphabetical order below.

▸ **AIDSDRUGS** covers HIV and AIDS from 1980 to the present. It is free through HealthGate at: http://www.healthgate.com/.
▸ **AIDSLINE** covers references on HIV and AIDS from 1980. It is free through HealthGate at: http://www.healthgate.com/.
▸ **AIDSTRIALS** covers trials of HIV and AIDS from 1980 to the present. It is free through HealthGate at: http://www.healthgate.com/.
▸ **AMED** (Allied and Alternative Medicine) is a unique database, only available on CD-ROM via OVID, that searches across the spectrum of complementary and alternative medicine. It covers reference articles from 400 journals, many of which are not indexed elsewhere, from 1985 to the present. For more information see http://minos.bl.uk/services/stb/amed.html.
▸ **ASSIA plus** (Applied Social Sciences Index and Abstracts) covers all major social sciences and related media including sociology, social policy, psychology and relevant aspects of anthropology, economics, medicine, law and politics. It features over 215 000 records from over 600 English

language journals, covering 16 countries, including 25 of the 30 most cited sources. It covers the period since 1987 and is updated quarterly. It is produced by Bowker Saur and is available on CD-ROM. For more information see their website: http://www.bowker-saur.co.uk/products/catalog/a_and_i/assia_plus_c.htm.

▶ **Best Evidence** provides commentaries from abstracts that have been published in the *ACP Journal Club* and *Evidence Based Medicine* journals which provide detailed abstracts from published studies and reviews from 1991. It includes assessments of quality by clinical experts. It is updated annually and is simple to use, but provides incomplete coverage of the literature. It is available as a yearly subscription on CD-ROM from the BMJ Publishing Group (0207 387 4499) and at: http://hiru.hirunet.mcmaster.ca/acpjc.

▶ **BIOETHICSLINE** covers bio-ethical literature from 1973 onwards, including newspaper articles, books and court judgements. It is free through HealthGate at: http://www.healthgate.com/.

▶ **CANCERLIT** covers the treatment of cancer and information on epidemiology, pathogenesis and immunology from 1976 to date. It is free through HealthGate at: http://www.healthgate.com/.

▶ **East Anglia University** has a database for midwives that will especially suit those new to searching the web. You can find it at: http://www.uea.ac.uk/~x645.

▶ **EDINA BIOSIS** covers more than 6500 articles from more than 90 countries from 1985 to the present. It covers biological sciences and related subjects, including public health. It is updated every two weeks and over 500 000 articles are added annually. EDINA offers the UK tertiary education and research community networked access to a library of data, information and research resources. All EDINA services are available free of charge to members of UK tertiary education institutions for academic use. Institutional subscription and personal registration is required for most services. It is available at: http://edina.ed.ac.uk/about.html.

▶ **ENB Health Care Database Search** is the English National Board (ENB) for Nursing, Midwifery and Health Visiting search facility. This database includes abstracts of over 4000 citations from the main UK and American journals. It is at: http://www.enb.org.uk/cgi-bin/hcdsearch. This website may change after September 2001 when the National Boards are disbanded following changes to the nursing, midwifery and health visiting statutory bodies. Try UKCC sites for further directions.

▶ **PsycINFO**® includes worldwide literature from 1967 to the present in the field of psychology and psychological aspects of related disciplines, including medicine, psychiatry, nursing, sociology, education, pharmacology, physiology, linguistics, anthropology, business and law. PsycINFO® is updated monthly and covers 1300 journals in 25 languages – over 45 000 references are added annually. Searching and browsing titles is free. It is available at: http://www.healthgate.com/.

▶ **PsycLIT**® is the electronic version of *Psychological Abstracts* produced by the American Psychological Association. It contains 1 000 000+ records from over 45 countries in more than 30 languages covering psychology and related disciplines such as medicine, psychiatry, education, nursing, social science and pharmacology. PsycLIT indexes around 1300 international journals, plus dissertations, book chapters, books, technical reports and other documents from 1974 for journals and 1987 for books. It is available on CD-ROM and is updated quarterly.

▶ **SUMSearch** is a new method for searching the Internet for EBM information. It queries a variety of databases including Medline, the Merck Manual, the National Guideline Clearinghouse from the Agency for Health Care Policy and Research (AHCPR), PubMed and DARE. SUMSearch automatically corrects common abbreviations and common terms that are hard to search for on common databases. For example, it converts *DVT* to *deep vein thrombosis* and *heart failure* to *heart failure or ventricular failure* – small changes that greatly affect Medline. It is available free at: http://SUMsearch.uthscsa.edu.

Other information on the Internet [24,25]

- ▸ **Bath Information and Data Service (BIDS)**[19] at http://www.bids.ac.uk is a database designed to be used by non-expert searchers and includes several medically orientated databases such as Embase, Citation Indexes, and Inside Information, with a wide variety of medically related reference material.
- ▸ **Health on the Net** at http://www.hon.ch. The Health on the Net Foundation has developed a code of conduct for medical and health websites. This states that medical information should either be given by medically trained and qualified professionals or, if this is not possible, it should be indicated clearly that the information is given by non-medically qualified people. Websites complying with this code bear the Health on the Net logo. But the presence of a logo is not a guarantee of the quality of the information.
- ▸ The **Health Technology Assessment (HTA)** programme is a national programme of research established and funded by the Department of Health's Research Programme: http://www.hta.nhsweb.nhs.uk. Health Technology Assessments are peer reviewed, rapid systematic reviews, cost effectiveness analyses of health interventions and technologies which are produced by several groups.
- ▸ **Medical Matrix** at http://www.medmatrix.org. This data base is published by Healthtel Corp., with around 4000 quality-assessed Internet sites of clinical medicine topics ranked for quality.
- ▸ Accessing databases of published research is easy. However, accessing information on research in progress is more difficult. The **National Research Register (NRR)** is a register of ongoing or recently completed research and development projects funded by, or of interest to, the NHS. It also contains details of reviews in progress collected by the NHS Centre for Reviews and Dissemination (CRD). The current release contains information on over 57 000 research projects, as well as entries from the Medical Research Council's Clinical Trials Register. The NRR is

assembled and published by Update Software Ltd on behalf of the Department of Health in the United Kingdom. The complete NRR database is free on the Internet at http://www.doh.gov.uk/research/nrr.htm. It is also available on CD-ROM at local health research libraries. Further information is available from: The NRR Project Administrator, NHS Executive Headquarters, Research & Development Directorate, Room 5W34, Quarry House, Quarry Hill, Leeds LS2 7UE.

► **PubMed** is the National Library of Medicine's search service that was developed in conjunction with publishers of biomedical literature as a search tool for accessing literature citations and linking to full-text journals at websites of participating publishers. It provides access to over 11 000 000 citations in Medline, PreMedline (updated daily and provides basic citation information and abstracts before the citation is indexed and added to Medline), HealthSTAR and other related databases, with links to participating online journals. Although PubMed is free, user registration, a subscription fee, or a fee may be required to access the full text of articles in some journals. It is available at http://www.ncbi.nlm.nih.gov/PubMed/

► The **'NEW' TRIP** database is a one-stop search engine for evidence-based material on the Internet. It is an amalgamation of 26 databases of hyperlinks from 'evidence-based' sites around the world. There are currently over 10 000 links to evidence-based topics. It is available at http://www.tripdatabase.com/

Website for learning evidence-based medicine skills[26]

EBM at McMaster University at http://hiru.hirunet.mcmaster.ca/ includes users' guides based on treatment and management of real cases.

Useful software

The Oxford Clinical Mentor[27] (OCM) is an electronic medical knowledge clinical support system developed by Oxford University Press with EMIS (Egton Medical Information Systems) practice computer systems. It has information about more than 2000 diseases cross-referenced with about 25 000 commonly used medical terms. The program comes up with a differential diagnosis for a set of symptoms, signs and test results, suggesting appropriate management plans which are a mix of evidence-based medicine and best practice. The information is regularly updated as new literature is published.

Electronic journals

All the titles listed below can be accessed free of charge. Some of the websites show the full contents of the journal, others do not carry the full text of all original articles.

► *British Medical Journal*
http://www.bmj.com
► *The Lancet*
http://www.thelancet.com

Full-text journals are also available free of charge from the American Medical Association at http://pubs.ama-assn.org/ Journals available include:

► *JAMA*
http://jama.ama-assn.org/
► *Archives of Dermatology*
http://archderm.ama-assn.org/issues/current/toc.html
► *Archives of Family Medicine*
http://archfami.ama-assn.org/issues/current/toc.html
► *Archives of Facial Plastic Surgery*
http://archfaci.ama-assn.org/issues/current/toc.html
► *Archives of Internal Medicine*
http://archinte.ama-assn.org/issues/current/toc.html

▶ *Archives of Pediatrics & Adolescent Medicine*
http://archpedi.ama-assn.org/issues/current/toc.html
▶ *Archives of Surgery*
http://archsurg.ama-assn.org/issues/current/toc.html
▶ *Archives of Neurology*
http://archneur.ama-assn.org/issues/current/toc.html
▶ *Archives of Ophthalmology*
http://archopht.ama-assn.org/issues/current/toc.html
▶ *Archives of Otolaryngology: Head & Neck Surgery*
http://archotol.ama-assn.org/issues/current/toc.html
▶ *Archives of General Psychiatry*
http://archpsyc.ama-assn.org/issues/current/toc.html

Nursing online journals

More and more journals are now available free and in full text online, and some electronic databases also give access to full text for some journals, so it is worth noting the ones that are relevant to you when carrying out a search.

▶ *British Journal of Midwifery*: you can subscribe to the online version of this journal at:
http://www.britishjournalofmidwifery.com. Annual subscription will cost around £65.
▶ *Nursing Standard On-Line*
http://www.nursing-standard.co.uk
▶ *Royal College of Midwives Journal*
http://www.midwives.co.uk and is free on the web.

The Free Medical Journals site is dedicated to the promotion of free access to medical journals over the Internet and is available at: http://www.freemedicaljournals.com/. This includes a selection of nursing and gynaecology journals, outlined below. The Free Medical Journals site also includes other journals from topic areas that may be relevant to midwifery, such as family planning, reproductive health, anaesthesiology, pain genetics and paediatrics.

▶ *Contemporary OB/GYN*
http://obgyn.pdr.net/obgyn/
▶ *Current Opinion in Obstetrics and Gynecology*
http://www.co-obgyn.com/
▶ *Journal Watch Women's Health*
http://www.jwatch.org/wh/
▶ *Journal of Community Nursing*
http://www.jcn.co.uk/
▶ *Nursing Spectrum*
http://www.nursingspectrum.com/
▶ *Nursing Standard*
http://www.nursing-standard.co.uk/
▶ *Obstetrics and Gynaecology Communications*
http://www.scientific-com.com/ObsGynCom/
▶ *Online Journal of Issues in Nursing*
http://www.nursingworld.org/ojin/

> **'The greatest obstacle to discovering the truth is being convinced that
> you already know it.'**

Useful websites for midwives

▶ MIDIRS (Midwives Information and Resource Service)

MIDIRS provides up-to-date information on any aspect of midwifery, childbirth and maternity care, and lists details of relevant Internet resource sites. It is available on the Internet at www.midirs.org and membership costs £42 per annum for a UK student on a bursary and £54 per annum for UK midwives (2001 prices). This gives you:

- unlimited online access to over 300 MIDIRS standard searches
- unlimited online access to the MIDIRS database for non-standard enquiry searches (over 76 000 references to original articles)

- the quarterly journal MIDIRS Midwifery Digest, delivered by post. The material in the Digest comes from a wide range of sources. MIDIRS scans over 550 journals in the search for new information. The articles that are most interesting and relevant are then selected for inclusion in the Midwifery Digest. MIDIRS' daily news articles cover current issues of the day and provide interesting links/files. You also receive regular e-mail updates on the topic of your choice.
- electronic midwifery news, information, forthcoming events and access to the online resource centre
- a new MIDIRS member certificate.

The MIDIRS library stocks all the journal articles and most of the books and reports included on MIDIRS, so, copyright laws permitting, they can send you a photocopy of the information you need. Contact MIDIRS at: 9 Elmdale Road, Clifton, Bristol BS8 1SL. Tel: 0800 581 009 (UK only); Fax: 0117 925 1792.

There are a number of other useful websites that are designed to help nurses, midwives and other healthcare professionals to link up with relevant resources on the Internet. These are outlined below.

The National Boards provide a range of practice information about midwifery, research and development, policy documents, programmes of nursing, midwifery education and much more.

▶ The English National Board (ENB) for Nursing, Midwifery and Health Visiting is on the web at:
http://www.enb.org.uk/
▶ The National Board for Nursing, Midwifery and Health Visiting for Scotland is at:
http://www.nbs.org.uk/
▶ The National Board for Nursing, Midwifery and Health Visiting for Northern Ireland is at:
http://www.n-i.nhs.uk/NBNI/

▸ The Welsh National Board for Nursing, Midwifery and Health Visiting is at:
http://www.wnb.org.uk/

▸ The United Kingdom Central Council (UKCC) is an organisation set up by Parliament to ensure that nurses, midwives and health visitors provide high standards of care to their patients and clients. It is at:
http://www.ukcc.org.uk/cms/content/home/

▸ OMNI offers free access to a searchable catalogue of Internet sites covering health and medicine, including midwifery. It is free on the web at:
http://omni.ac.uk/

▸ Midwifery Links lists sites of interest to midwives and is at:
http://www.qmced.ac.uk/lb/www/links/midwife.htm

▸ Nursing and Health Care Resources on the Net at the University of Sheffield is designed to help nurses, midwives and other healthcare professionals to link up with resources on the Net. From Spring 2001 it is at:
http://nmahp.ac.uk

▶ STAGE 1

Asking the right question[28]

Although you may be burning to ask your question, when you actually try to set it down on paper, you may find that the exercise is more difficult than you think.

Questions have to be phrased in a very specific way to obtain meaningful responses in any context. This applies to asking other people what they think about a topic as much as to searching the literature for the best evidence.

The best clinical questions relate to queries arising from your own patients during the course of your work rather than being hypothetical questions. Relevant work-based questions should motivate you to seek the evidence and make change(s). Before you go to a lot of trouble to find answers or solutions to your questions, ask around at work and find out if anyone else is concerned about the same question or problem, already has the answer(s), or knows where to find them.

The question should be:

▶ simple
▶ specific
▶ realistic
▶ important
▶ capable of being answered
▶ agreed and owned by those who will be involved in any changes resulting
▶ implementable
▶ about a topic where change will be possible.

Think about how to construct your clinical question by considering:

▶ what the question is about. For example, is the question about an individual or a group of patients? What are the patient characteristics you are interested in, such as age or parity? Is it a clinical dilemma or a resource problem?
▶ the setting. For example, is it specific to rural or urban locations?
▶ the type of intervention and whether it is being compared with current practice or another intervention. For example, are you interested in different approaches to care or risk assessment, compared with current practice or no intervention?
▶ the outcome(s) of the clinical topic. For example, is an acceptable outcome to your question a decrease in the uptake of antenatal screening or better informed consent?

You should focus and phrase your question to include whatever it is that you want to know about effects, efficiency, outcome of an intervention or user satisfaction. You may decide to have a main question with several subsidiary questions.

Questions about cost-effectiveness

'Cost-effective' is not synonymous with 'cheap'.

A cost-effective intervention is one which gives a better or equivalent benefit from the intervention in question for lower or equivalent cost, or where the relative improvement in outcome is higher than the relative difference in cost. In other words, being cost-effective means having the best outcomes for the least input. Using the term 'cost-effective' implies that you have considered potential alternatives.

An intervention must first be considered *clinically* effective to warrant investigation into its potential to be *cost*-effective. Evidence-based practice must incorporate clinical judgement. You have to interpret the evidence when it comes to applying it to individual patients, whether it be evidence about clinical effectiveness or about cost-effectiveness.

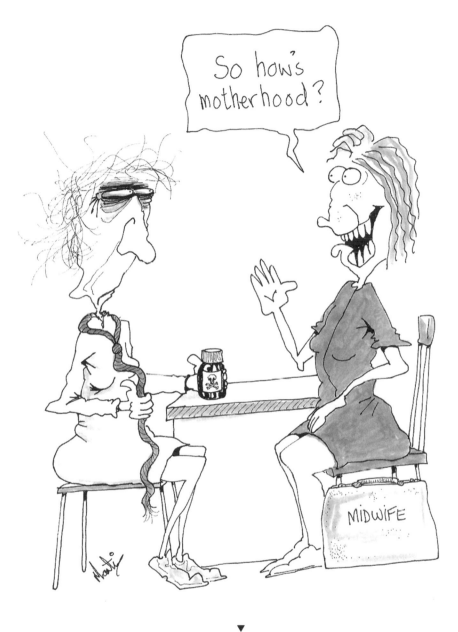

▼
Asking inappropriate questions.

If you want to ask a question about cost-effectiveness you should be sure to have confirmed clinical effectiveness first, and have gone on to ask a question about cost-effectiveness as the second stage in seeking the evidence.

A 'benefit' is what is gained from meeting a chosen need and a 'cost' is the benefit that would have been obtained from using the same resources in an alternative way. Opportunity costs are the costs of the benefits foregone in deploying resources in the chosen way.

A new or alternative intervention should be compared directly with the next best intervention.

An economic evaluation is a comparative analysis of two or more alternatives in terms of their costs and consequences.[29] There are four different types: cost-effectiveness, cost minimisation, cost–utility analysis and cost–benefit analysis. Cost-effectiveness analysis is used to compare the effectiveness of two interventions with the same treatment objectives. Cost minimisation compares the costs of alternative interventions which have identical health outcomes. Cost–utility analysis enables the effects of alternative interventions to be measured against a combination of life expectancy and quality of life, a common outcome measure being 'quality-adjusted life-years' (QALYs). A cost–benefit analysis compares the incremental costs and benefits of a programme.

Efficiency is sometimes confused with effectiveness. Being efficient means having obtained the most quality from the least expenditure, or the required level of quality for the least expenditure. To measure efficiency you need to make a judgement about the level of quality of the 'purchase' and be able to relate it to 'price'. 'Price' alone does not measure efficiency. Quality is the indicator used in combination with price to assess whether something is more efficient.

So, cost-effectiveness is a measure of efficiency and suggests that costs have been related to effectiveness.

'I have finally made up my mind but the decision was by no means unanimous.'

Framing questions: some examples

Now try these two examples of clinical situations and frame a specific question for each with which you might search the literature for evidence to answer the question.

Jot down notes under each heading and write the final question at the bottom of the page ready to do a trial literature search using the Medline database. Refine and limit the question to what would seem to be a relevant question for midwives delivering maternity services. Your question should be shaped by thinking out exactly why you are asking it and how you might apply the evidence in practice once you have obtained it.

Set a question to address problem 1

An antenatal clinic is taking stock of the preventive work it does and is reviewing whether to continue the range of work that different health professionals offer. The community midwives and other staff are wondering what the impact is of the range of health education about smoking that they offer their patients.

1 What is the question about – an individual patient, a group of people, a particular population, patient characteristics, a clinical dilemma, a resource problem?

2 What is the setting or context of the clinical topic/situation?

3 Is there an intervention and, if so, with what is it being compared?

4 What is/are the outcome(s) of the clinical topic?

5 What is the specific question you will ask?

6 Choose up to four key words, in priority order, that you think best represent the important components of your question and that will restrict it as far as possible to your field of enquiry.

Some example details follow.

Example details of question posed to address problem 1

Defining the question

The refined question should narrow down the limits of the enquiry by specifying as many of the following details as apply:

► What is the question about – the whole or a section of the practice population? What is meant by health education? Which staff are involved with the health education intervention? What is meant by 'smoking', etc.?
► What is the setting or context of the enquiry? The focus of your interest might be antenatal care, postnatal care or the impact of smoking on the neonate.
► Is there an intervention and, if so, with what is it being compared? What types of health education is the questioner interested in? Is there an alternative model to which health education is being compared?

> ► What is/are the outcome(s) of the health education intervention and what is meant by 'impact'? e.g. changes in attitudes, quantity of cigarettes smoked, reduction in detriment to health.
> ► The specific question will have narrowed down the problem to one in which the midwives are interested. For instance, if midwives were reviewing whether to continue the pre-conception clinic, besides looking at attendance figures, patient preferences, and opportunity costs for staff, the midwives might want to know 'what is the evidence for the effectiveness of face-to-face education about the risks of cigarette smoking in midwife-run clinics?' A more general question might be 'what is the evidence for the effectiveness of a health professional advising a smoker to stop smoking?'
> ► Key words might be *health education*, *smoking*, *maternity*, etc. depending on your question. You might have other key words.

Comments from participants' experiences at the live workshops on clinical effectiveness

Participants found that each small group composed entirely different questions as they had different foci of interests. Some found that their question did not contain the key words they selected after finalising their question, as they had not refined their ideas sufficiently. The result was that in some cases a later search on the chosen key words on Medline missed the point of the question.

Set a question to address problem 2

A pregnant woman asks her midwife if she should try acupuncture for her early morning sickness and if it will reduce her constant nausea.

Have a go at completing parts of the question for problem 2:

1 What is the question about – an individual patient, a group of people, a particular population, patient characteristics, a clinical dilemma, a resource problem?

2 What is the setting or context of the clinical topic/situation?

3 Is there an intervention and, if so, with what is it being compared?

4 What is/are the outcome(s) of the clinical topic?

5 What is the specific question you will ask?

6 Choose up to four key words in priority order that you think best represent the important components of your question and that will restrict them as far as possible to your field of enquiry.

Some example details follow.

Example details of question posed to address problem 2

Defining the question

A refined question will narrow down the limits of the enquiry by specifying as many of the following details as apply:

- ▶ What is the question about – the woman or all pregnant women suffering from morning sickness, e.g. nausea, vomiting or both? What is meant by morning sickness? What is meant by acupuncture?
- ▶ What is the setting or context of the enquiry? The focus of your interest might be antenatal clinics, the community or primary care.
- ▶ If there is an intervention, with what is it being compared – the method of acupuncture, or any other type of intervention for morning sickness?
- ▶ What is/are the outcome(s) of the intervention and what is meant by *reduce* – changes in nausea symptoms, reduction in frequency of vomiting?
- ▶ The specific question should narrow down the problem to one in which the woman and midwife are interested. So you might ask 'what is the evidence for the effectiveness of acupuncture point stimulation in controlling nausea and vomiting associated with morning sickness?'
- ▶ Key words might be *acupuncture, nausea, morning sickness, pregnancy.* You might have other key words.

Examples of questions midwives might pose from their everyday practice

These are questions you might use to search for the evidence, and when you find the evidence, interpret it and decide whether or not to put that evidence into practice.

There are some questions for which there is little evidence, where an expert opinion is the best available evidence. There are other questions where we have evidence from randomised controlled trials and systematic reviews, such as those below.[30]

▶ What are the effects of routine ultrasound screening?

The evidence: 'Routine ultrasound screening before 24 weeks gestation leads to: (i) earlier diagnosis of multiple pregnancies but has not been shown to have an important positive impact on the outcome of multiple pregnancies; (ii) fewer inductions of labour for 'post-term' pregnancy; (iii) generally high rates of detection of abnormalities on the central nervous system, and low rates of detection of skeletal and cardiac abnormalities.'

▶ Is routine Doppler ultrasound of the umbilical or uterine arteries beneficial in unselected or low-risk pregnancies?

The evidence: 'Doppler ultrasound in pregnancy has not been shown to be of benefit, and may even increase the risk of adverse outcome.'

▶ Does midline episiotomy incision have the same outcome as mediolateral incision?

The evidence: There is 'no evidence that midline episiotomy incision improves outcome compared with mediolateral incision. Limited evidence suggests that midline incision may increase the risk of third and fourth degree tears'.

▶ Is perineal trauma more common in an upright position compared with a recumbent position during delivery?

The evidence: One systematic review found 'no significant difference in overall rates of perineal trauma'. A subsequent randomised controlled trial found a reduced episiotomy rate, a slight increase in labial trauma, and slight reduction in third degree tears in women who delivered in an upright position.

▶ What are the effects of different methods and materials for primary repair of perineal trauma, including non-suturing?

The evidence: 'The use of absorbable synthetic suture materials with a continuous subcuticular stitch to appose the skin reduces short-term pain. The effects on long-term pain and other complications remain uncertain.' There is 'no evidence that leaving the perineal skin unsutured alters short-term pain, but dysparunia is reduced at three months postpartum'.

▸ What are the effects of preventive interventions in women at high risk of pre-eclampsia?

The evidence: 'Anti-platelet drugs (mainly aspirin) reduce the risk of pre-eclampsia ... calcium supplementation reduces the relative risk of pre-eclampsia by about a third.' There is 'insufficient evidence on the effects of fish oil, or of evening primrose oil plus fish oil or calcium on the risk of pre-eclampsia and preterm birth'.

▸ What are the effects of interventions in women who develop hypertension in pregnancy?

The evidence: There is 'limited evidence from which it is not possible to demonstrate benefit for hospital admission, bed rest or day care compared with outpatient care'. ... 'It is unclear whether women with mild to moderate hypertension during pregnancy derive benefit from antihypertensive drugs.' ... 'For women with severe hypertension during pregnancy, antihypertensive drugs will lower blood pressure.' There is 'promising evidence that magnesium sulphate may reduce the risk of developing eclampsia, but other possible benefits and harms are unclear'.

▸ What is the best choice of anticonvulsant for women with eclampsia?

The evidence: 'Magnesium sulphate is the best choice of anticonvulsant for treatment of eclampsia.'

▸ What are the effects of preventive interventions in women at high risk of preterm delivery?

The evidence: 'Antibiotic treatment of bacterial vaginosis during pregnancy decreases the incidence of preterm delivery, especially in women who have had a previous preterm delivery.' There is no evidence that 'enhanced antenatal care reduces the risk of preterm delivery'. In women 'presumed to have cervical incompetence, cervical cerclage is associated with a significant reduction in preterm births (less than 33 weeks gestation)'.

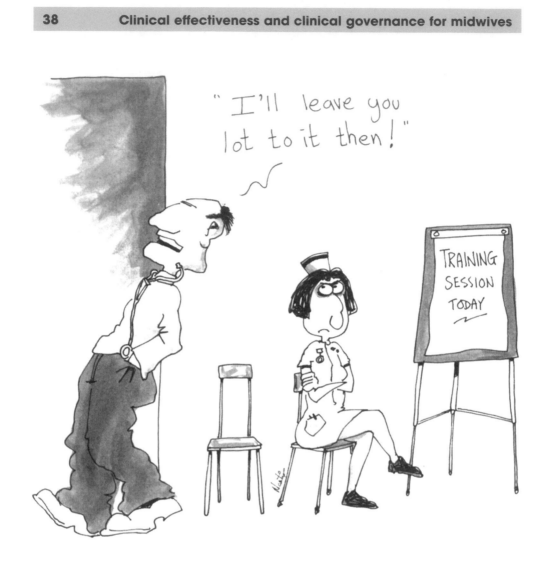

Clinical effectiveness is done best by involving the whole team.

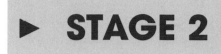

► STAGE 2

Undertaking a library search

The search strategy: think, search and appraise

A search for the best evidence follows the sequence of 'think, search and appraise'. This search strategy comprises:

► thinking about and defining a good specific question in consultation with all the staff who are involved in the question and affected by possible change(s)
► searching for and finding the best level of evidence by looking critically at the relevant publications obtained
► appraising and interpreting the evidence as applied to your question in relation to your situation.

Clinical effectiveness encompasses the whole cycle:

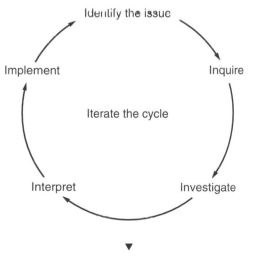

The clinical effectiveness cycle.

It is tempting for health professionals who are rushed for time and hot on the scent of evidence to a question to jump straight from an idea to carrying out a search, instead of working through the steps with the necessary rigour. Cutting corners wastes time in the long run if you ask the wrong question, answer a different question to the one you intended, or become distracted by lots of interesting but irrelevant literature.

How long you spend and to what lengths you go with a search will depend on its purpose. If you were commissioned to undertake a major systematic review, you would spend many months searching every relevant database, hand searching through papers and journals, hunting up conference proceedings, trying personal contacts, translating non-English language papers, and generally leaving no stone unturned in the pursuit of published and unpublished studies. But as you are probably a busy midwife who just wants to find the best evidence for answering a question in practice, you should strictly limit your search, as your resources are limited. You will probably be better off spending your precious time doing several searches for different topics than doing one exhaustive search on a single subject. So stop your search as soon as you find a relevant systematic review of multiple, well-designed, randomised controlled trials in the Cochrane database. If there is no such systematic review in the Cochrane database move on to look for a review in the Database of Abstracts of Effectiveness Reviews (DARE). If no luck there, try Medline, or Embase or other specialist databases until you obtain the best possible level of evidence that you can find.

If you have not undertaken a search of the literature before, you would be well advised to book an individual session with your local university health librarian and to undertake a search in your postgraduate medical library if this is possible. You should be able to teach yourself from guidebooks, these notes, and trial and error, but a specialist librarian is the person with the know-how about the best terms and phrases to try with your search. You will know about the validity, context and relevance of search words and phrases as applied to your question. Together, you as a midwife and the medical librarian make a strong search team.

Look back at the database, website and online journal details we described earlier on – MIDIRS might be especially useful.

Undertake a search

Before you start *write down* the key words you want to use and prioritise their order of importance. How many key words you enter as the first stage depends on how wide you expect your field of enquiry to be. If you key in *breast feeding* you would expect to identify thousands more references to published papers than if you keyed in the name of a rare condition. So if you are searching within a broad topic area such as *breast feeding* you should prepare more potential words to narrow the field of your search for the few most relevant papers that will supply evidence to answer your original question. Refine your question prior to your search so that it is very focused and make sure that the key words are the most pertinent you can manage. Then you will spend less time on your search and have more chance of finding the most appropriate published evidence. So if you want to know more in the subject area of *breast feeding*, build your question carefully. Aim specifically at the purpose of the question and include the setting, the population under question, the intervention, the outcome and any other important details.

In order to help in the search for evidence, a number of pre-defined search strategies have been published. These are a tailored set of instructions for locating randomised controlled trials (RCTs), systematic reviews, meta-analyses etc. Systematic reviews on Medline and CINAHL can be found at http://www.york.ac.uk/inst/crd/search.htm. Other search strategies including those for RCTs are available at http://www.ncbi.nlm.nih.gov/PubMed/clinical.html.

Using the Cochrane database

Enter your most important key words first – perhaps two words, as there are relatively few publications on the Cochrane database compared to other databases. Look at the different levels of evidence from the systematic reviews on the Cochrane Database of Systematic Reviews (CDSR), to controlled trials on the Cochrane Controlled Trials Register (CCTR), to the abstracts on the Database of Abstracts of Reviews of Effectiveness (DARE). The hierarchy of evidence is explained further in the next section.

It is likely that you will obtain only a small number of references to relevant-sounding systematic reviews because, as mentioned above, the Cochrane has relatively few publications on its databases in comparison to others. It is more likely that you will not find a relevant systematic review, but will identify many references to controlled trials. You should then modify your search further by entering the first two key words again plus a third key word that was your next choice in priority order in your original list of key words constructed prior to beginning your search. If this has not refined your search enough, repeat the exercise, adding a fourth key word. When you have narrowed your search sufficiently, print off the abstracts of the papers you have identified and obtain copies of the original articles as appropriate so that you can critically appraise them yourself.

Do not assume that the contents of any paper published in a journal are valid, reliable or accurate, however reputable the journal. Mistakes may have been overlooked, studies reported might not be relevant to your own situation, or the results may not be generalisable to your question.

If your search on the Cochrane database has been unsuccessful, move on to another database which has many more references to medical publications, such as Medline.

Using the Medline database

Because Medline has a phenomenal number of references you will have to develop a very strict search strategy to narrow down your focus of enquiry. To operate a search on Medline, you can use the key words that occur in its thesaurus of medical terms, the medical subject heading list (MeSH). There are over 17500 MeSH terms arranged as a tree structure with broad subject areas branching off and sub-dividing into narrower subject terms. If you key in a word which is not a MeSH term, Medline will give you a choice of terms with close meanings. For instance if you key in 'cigarettes', which is not a key word in MeSH, Medline will give you 'smoking', 'smoking cessation' or 'cannabis smoking' as alternative words or phrases.

You can trace published literature on Medline by either searching for your own key word(s) in the title, abstract, author's name, or body of any articles or papers, or by searching for articles containing selected words from the MeSH list.

Entering one key word will often yield thousands of references to published articles. So, you can do a more selective search by combining key words using the instructions 'and' and 'or' (these are called Boolean operators). To narrow the search further you can specify the numbers of years of literature searched, the language the paper is written in, the papers in the journals of the abridged *Index Medicus*, and 'human' as opposed to 'animal' research.

In a university library, all you will need to do to access Medline and the Cochrane databases is to click on the icons on your screen, signposting you to the relevant databases. You may use Ovid software or another standard communications programme to access the Medline service.

There are two publications giving easy-to-follow practical details of undertaking a Medline search[31] which you could consult if you are unfamiliar with Medline searching and want to read more about the process before having a go for yourself.

Hints for the use of Medline (adapted from Ovid Technologies software) are:

▶ click on a **Subject Heading** to view its tree of key words or terms
▶ select the **Explode** box to retrieve references using your selected key word and all the more specific terms stemming from it
▶ select the **Focus** box to limit your search to those documents in which your key word (subject heading) is considered to be the main point of the article
▶ if the topic of your search does not map to a desirable subject heading, click on the box **Search as Keyword**.

You will learn most by having a go. You really cannot do anything wrong that you are not able to put right by retracing your steps. There are help boxes and icons throughout the database forms.

The hierarchy of evidence

The table below shows the generally agreed strengths of evidence ranging from level I, which is the most robust evidence, to level V based on the opinions of experts in the field.[28] But there may not be any evidence in the literature for answering the question(s) you are posing.

Type	Evidence
I	Strong evidence from at least one systematic review of multiple, well-designed, randomised controlled trials
II	Strong evidence from at least one properly designed, randomised controlled trial of appropriate size
III	Evidence from well-designed trials without randomisation, single group pre–post, cohort, time series or matched case–control studies
IV	Evidence from well-designed non-experimental studies from more than one centre or research group
V	Opinions of respected authorities, based on clinical evidence, descriptive studies or reports of expert committees

The most valid types of research for extracting evidence about clinical effectiveness are randomised controlled trials, followed by controlled trials, then trials and, less reliably, observational studies. A systematic review of several randomised controlled studies or all known studies is better than a review of some studies, which in turn is better than a report of a case study. You should start to search for the best evidence and, if you do not find it, work down the hierarchy.

If there is no reliable evidence to be found after searching the Cochrane, Medline and other relevant databases, you should then move on to look for any expert consensus agreements by multidisciplinary groups.

Be realistic – try and find one or a few key reviews rather than get bogged down in a plethora of papers. Clinical effectiveness is a tool for keeping up to date with your clinical practice, retaining your professional interest and enhancing your effectiveness – spending too much time pursuing it may be counterproductive.

> 'Most of my problems either have no answer or else the answer is worse than the problem.'

Worked examples of undertaking a search

The Cochrane Library should be your first port of call when searching for research evidence. The usefulness of the Cochrane Library over and above Medline and CINAHL is demonstrated in the searches outlined below.

▶ Question 1: What is the evidence for the effectiveness of a midwife advising pregnant women to stop smoking?

Key words: *midwife, smoking, pregnancy*

Selected database: **Cochrane Database, 2000 Issue 4**

The Cochrane Database, 2000 Issue 4, was searched using the Advanced Search option. Searching for the MeSH heading *midwife* gives the term *Nurse-Midwives* and so this was chosen for the search. *Smoking cessation* was a branch of *smoking* and so this was chosen to help focus the search. *Pregnancy* was a MeSH term and was also chosen. These terms were then fed in one at a time to build up the search, the results of which are shown below.

Set	Search	Results
1	Smoking cessation*:ME	543
2	Pregnancy*:ME	39
3	(Combine) 1 and 2	39
4	Nurse-Midwives*:ME	37
5	Combine 3 and 4	1

This produced only one reference to a controlled trial on the Cochrane Controlled Trials Register (CCTR):

• Wakefield M and Jones W (1998) Effects of a smoking cessation programme for pregnant women and their partners attending a public hospital antenatal clinic. *Australian & New Zealand Journal of Public Health.* **22**(3): 313–20.

This seemed to be relevant to the question, but it only covered women with partners, and so the searcher moved on to search the **Ovid Medline Database <1997 to December 2000>**.

Midwife was not a MeSH term and so *Midwifery* was used instead. *Smoking cessation* is a branch of *smoking* and so was chosen to restrict the search. The results are outlined in the table opposite. Sets 1 and 2 show how many papers, published from 1997 onwards, were held by Medline where *midwifery* or *smoking cessation* were listed on the database. The 'explode' command was chosen to avoid restricting the search to a subsection of the Medline database 'tree' and to allow the searcher to access all possible articles on Medline. Using the explode function avoids relying on the MeSH indexer, with whose categorisation you may not agree. Combining sets 1 and 2 resulted in a set 3 with only two studies and so it was not necessary to include *pregnancy* in the search.

Set	Search	Results
1	Explode Midwifery/	557
2	Explode Smoking cessation/	1812
3	(Combine) 1 and 2	2

The two studies that the search revealed did appear to address the question: one was carried out in Denmark (Wisborg *et al.*, 1998) and the other in the USA (Klerman and Rooks, 1999). So the searcher moved on to search CINAHL to see if there was any evidence from research carried out in a British setting that might be more generalisable to midwives in the UK.

- Klerman LV and Rooks JP (1999) A simple, effective method that midwives can use to help pregnant women stop smoking. *Journal of Nurse-Midwifery.* **44**(2): 118–23.
- Wisborg K, Henriksen TB and Secher NJ (1998) A prospective intervention study of stopping smoking in pregnancy in a routine antenatal care setting. *British Journal of Obstetrics and Gynaecology.* **105**(11): 1171–6.

Ovid allows the database to be changed and gives the option of repeating the search strategy. Thus, the Medline search was repeated using **Ovid CINAHL<1996 to November 2000>**.

Set	Search	Results
1	Explode Midwifery/	1774
2	Explode Smoking cessation/	812
3	(Combine) 1 and 2	8

The search strategy this time revealed eight studies and the abstracts of all eight suggested that they were relevant. Only one of these studies (Arborelius and Nyberg, 1997) was set outside the UK.

- Arborelius E and Nyberg K (1997) How should midwives discuss smoking behaviour in pregnancy with women of low educational attainment? *Midwifery.* **13**(4): 210–15.

It is interesting that the studies by Klerman and Rooks (1999) and Wisborg *et al.* (1998) identified by the Medline search were not revealed by the CINAHL search, and that the Wakefield and Jones (1998) paper that the Cochrane Library revealed did not appear in either the Medline or the CINAHL search. This is probably due to the fact that different databases include different journals, and highlights the need to search more than one database.

▶ Question 2: What is the evidence for the effectiveness of the external cephalic version for breech presentation at term?

Key words: *breech presentation, fetal version*

Selected database: **The Cochrane Database, 2000 Issue 4**

Keying in *breech* into the MeSH headings gave the terms *breech presentation* and *fetal version*. These were fed in one at a time to build up the search as outlined in the table below.

Set	Search	Results
1	Breech presentation*:ME	47
2	Version-fetal*:ME	33
3	(Combine) 1 and 2	28

Combining sets 1 and 2 gave a total of 28 hits, three of which were on the Cochrane Database of Systematic Reviews (CDSR). These were all updates of one systematic review and the latest substantive amendment, made in 1997, is referenced here (Hofmeyr, 2000).

• Hofmeyr GJ (2000) External cephalic version facilitation for breech presentation at term (Cochrane Review). *The Cochrane Library*, Issue 4, Update Software, Oxford.

The remaining 25 hits were made on the Cochrane Controlled Trials Register (CCTR). No hits were made on the Database of Abstracts of Reviews of Effectiveness (DARE) or on the NHS Economic Evaluation Database (NHS EED). Browsing through the trials, 21 seemed to be relevant to the question.

The searcher then moved on to select the **Medline Database <1997 to December 2000>**. The search strategy used the MeSH terms *breech presentation* and *fetal version*, fed in one at a time to build up the search. The terms were exploded to ensure full coverage.

Set	Search	Results
1	Explode breech presentation/	186
2	Explode version, fetal/	78
3	(Combine) 1 and 2	45
4	Limit 3 to English language	40
5	Limit 4 to review articles	7

Combining sets 1 and 2 gave 45 studies, which was considered too many to look at, and so set 4 confined the references obtained in set 3 to the 40 publications that were written in English. Forty articles were still considered to be too many abstracts to browse through; so in order to limit the search further, the searcher limited set 4 to review articles only, which gave seven. Reading the abstracts revealed that all seven were relevant to the question.

To see if there was any other evidence available, the searcher then transferred the same search to **CINAHL<1996 to November 2000>**.

Set	Search	Results
1	Explode breech presentation/	81
2	Explode version, fetal/	15
3	(Combine) 1 and 2	12
4	Limit 3 to English language	12
5	Limit 4 to review articles	0

There were no review articles and limiting the set to English language did not reduce the number of articles. However, it was realistic to scroll through the 12 articles in set 4, nine of which appeared to be relevant to the question.

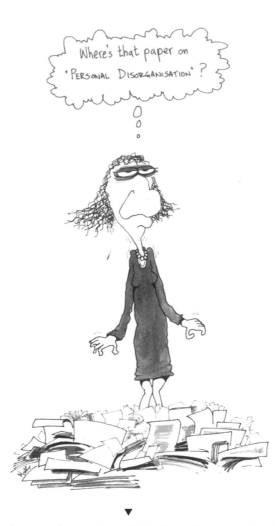

▼

Use IT to ask a question and search for the evidence systematically.

Additional tips for undertaking a search

▶ To reduce your reliance on the indexers and minimise your chances of missing any papers relevant to your search that the indexer might have categorised differently from how you expected, you should employ a 'belt and braces' technique. For instance, if your question is about screening for a disease, you may find that keying in *screen$.tw* identifies any article on the database where *screen, screening* or *screens* is used as a textword (tx in Cochrane, tw in Medline and CINAHL) in the abstract.

▸ MeSH terms might not identify all relevant studies. For example, the MeSH term *Breast Neoplasms* identified 2613 references in the Cochrane Library. Putting a phrase in inverted commas ensures that it is searched as a phrase and when *'Breast Neoplasm' and* was searched as a textword using the 'Advanced Search' option this produced 3143 references.

▸ In the first search described above, *smoking cessation* was chosen to help focus the search as it is a branch of *smoking*. However, MeSH indexers sometimes get things wrong and so it might have been worth repeating the search using *smoking* to ensure that all relevant papers were identified.

▸ Keying in an umbrella term such as *diabet** (when your search question is focused on diabetes) can also be useful when searching. The asterisk (or wild card as it is known) ensures that words with slightly different endings such as *diabetic* and *diabetes* are included. For example, keying in *diabetes* revealed 6707 references, while keying in *diabet** revealed 8764 references. The symbol $ is used in Medline and CINAHL searches in place of the *.

▸ Searches can be narrowed further by adding another modification *aim*, which stands for 'Abridged *Index Medicus*', but these will include mainly American journals and by doing this you might miss UK-based publications.

▸ Another useful way of limiting a search is to see if your local searching facilities permit you to confine your search to 'local holdings' of literature, so that you can easily refer to original papers once you have identified the references from your computerised search.

You need to be aware that other countries might use different terms. For example, the USA might be more likely to use the term *family practice* than *primary healthcare*, which we use in the UK. Indeed, keying in and exploding *primary healthcare* produced 4878 hits while *family practice* produced 5543 hits (*family practice* was not exploded as it is at the end of a branch), and combining these using the term *or* produced 9864 papers. Thus, many of these publications would have been missed if only one of these terms had been used. Similarly, while *postnatal depression* is used widely in the UK, *postpartum depression* is used elsewhere, so both terms should be included for a comprehensive search strategy. You also need to be aware of different spellings of words and phrases, for example *fetal* and *foetal*, *labour* and *labor* and *caesarean* and *cesarean*. Some databases, such as SUMSearch, automatically search for both spellings, but others do not – so beware.

Searching by yourself

Now you do it – work through an example by yourself.

1 Take any one (or both) of the two problems which interests you most – whether health education on smoking is worth doing, or whether a breech presenting at term should be managed by external cephalic version. Adapt the problem(s) to your own circumstances. The idea of this exercise is that you will run a search on a question (or questions) similar to the ones already described so that you can follow the procedures laid out in this book for guidance, but adapted to your own situation so that it is more relevant to you. Conducting your own version of the search will give you more confidence that you can do a literature search yourself. Write in your own words what your perspective of the problem is:

2 Frame the words of your question to address that problem – the words you use in the question should vary from any

presented in this book, as the angle of the problem and the focus of the question should relate to your own circumstances. Write in your own words what the question is:

3 Choose up to five key words and put them in order of priority:

4 Undertake a search for the evidence to answer that problem. If possible go to your medical library and book time with a medical librarian and the computerised search facilities there. Use the Cochrane database first and then Medline.

Photocopy pages 52–5 if you undertake this exercise for more than one example question.

Cochrane search

▶ Write down how you will use your key words to search the Cochrane database. Which one, two or three words will you key in first? Then, which words will you add, and in what order, to narrow the focus of your search?

▶ How did the search go? How many 'hits' did you obtain from the Cochrane database?
  – systematic reviews on the Cochrane Database of Systematic Reviews (CDSR):
     (i) number of reviews =
     (ii) number of protocols =

     – controlled trials on the Cochrane Controlled Trials Register (CCTR) =
     – abstracts on the Database of Abstracts of Reviews of Effectiveness (DARE) =

► Write down up to five sets of details of articles that seem relevant to your question, giving article titles, authors' names, year of publication, volume of journal/source and page details so that you can obtain the original papers if you should wish to. Print off the abstracts if you have the facilities to do so.

Medline search

► Write down how you will use your key words to search the Medline database. Which one, two or three words will you key in first? Then, which words will you add, and in what order, to narrow the focus of your search?

► Begin your search and key the words in, exploding, combining and modifying the search according to the order of key words you have just specified and the numbers of papers you obtain at each stage. Go back to the instructions about using Medline and work through the examples and helpful suggestions if you have difficulties doing your own search.

► How did the search go? Print off the results of the search in the same way that the tables given as examples earlier listed the stages of the search, the modifications and the numbers of papers identified from the key words. If you cannot print the results off the screen, copy them down over the page under the sub-headings 'Set', 'Search' and 'Results' as in the example tables.

Set	Search	Results
1		

▶ When you get down to less than 20 or so articles, scroll through the abstracts on the screen and print off the details of the ones that seem most relevant. Write down up to five sets of details of articles that seem relevant, giving article titles, authors' names, year of publication, volume of journal/source and page details.

▶ If you have still not obtained any relevant evidence, you have a choice of trying other databases, or following up references given in papers with content nearest to your field of enquiry, or contacting experts named as authors or investigators to find out if there is work waiting to be published or other publications you have missed, or any other pertinent information.

You should not expect to find exactly the same details as in the examples given earlier. Not only will you have modified the problem, the linked question and the search strategy to fit your own circumstances, but the details of publications held on the Cochrane and Medline databases will have changed over time.

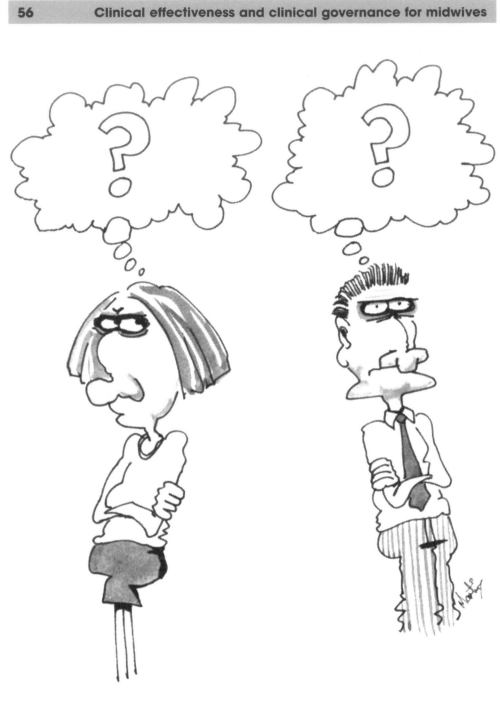

▼

Choose a question that is important to you and your colleagues at work and where changes in practice will be possible.

Frame your own question and search for the evidence

Now that you have learnt the theory behind doing a search and have seen how other health professionals like you have framed their questions and searched for the evidence, you should be ready to shape your own question and find the best available evidence that exists.

1 Think about a problem at work which you consider would be an appropriate topic for this exercise. Consult others at work: do they think it is a problem too? Is it an important issue for them and do they think you would be spending your time wisely searching for evidence about best practice? Is there likely to be a change that you could make which would bring benefits to you, colleagues or patients, or result in a saving of resources? As this book is considering how to improve clinical effectiveness, you should choose a clinical topic in this instance, but another time you might choose to search for evidence on a management issue. What is the problem you have chosen to investigate? Write it down here:

Who else did you consult before deciding on this problem?

What sort of changes at work do you have in mind that might be possible to put into action, depending on what evidence you find?

2 Frame the words of your question which address that problem. Build up the question as described previously, being as specific as possible, but not so specific that you narrow your field of enquiry and eliminate possible options that might be appropriate, such as novel types of interventions. Include the purpose of the question, what it is about, the setting, the population and the outcome(s). Write in your own words what the question is:

Are there any subsidiary questions?

Have you discussed the question with anyone else? If so, with whom?

3 Choose up to five key words and put them in order of priority:

Are you satisfied that these key words reflect all the essential ingredients of your original problem and capture the essence of the question?

4 Undertake a search for the evidence to answer the question. If possible go to your local university library and book time with an appropriate librarian and the computerised search facilities there. If the library has Cochrane and Medline searching facilities, try the Cochrane database first and then Medline.

Cochrane search

▶ Write down how you will use your key words to search the Cochrane database. Which one, two or three words will you key in first? Then, which words will you add, and in what order, to narrow the focus of your search?

▶ How did the search go? How many 'hits' did you obtain from the Cochrane database?
  – systematic reviews on the Cochrane Database of Systematic Reviews (CDSR):
    (i) number of reviews =
    (ii) number of protocols =
  – controlled trials on the Cochrane Controlled Trials Register (CCTR) =
  – abstracts on the Database of Abstracts of Reviews of Effectiveness (DARE) =

▶ Write down up to five sets of details of articles that seem relevant to your question, giving article titles, authors' names, year of publication, volume of journal/source and page details. Print off the abstracts of these articles if you are able to do so. Obtain copies of the original papers.

Medline search

▶ Write down how you will use your key words to search the Medline database. Which one, two or three words will you key in first? Then, which words will you add, and in what order, to narrow the focus of your search?

▶ Begin your search and key the words in, exploding, combining and modifying the search according to the order of key words you have just specified and the numbers of papers you obtain at each stage.

▶ How did the search go? Print off the results of the search in the same way that the tables given as examples earlier listed the stages of the search, the modifications and the numbers of papers identified from the key words. If you cannot print the results off the screen, copy them down here under the sub-headings 'Set', 'Search' and 'Results' as in the example tables.

Set	Search	Results
1		

▶ When you get down to less than 20 or so articles, scroll through the abstracts on the screen and print off the details of the ones that seem most relevant. Write down up to five sets of details of articles that seem relevant, giving article titles, authors' names, year of publication, volume of journal/ source and page details.

▶ If you have still not obtained any relevant evidence, you have a choice of trying other databases, or following up references given in papers with content nearest to your field of enquiry, or contacting experts named as authors or investigators to find out if there is work waiting to be published or other publications you have missed, or any other pertinent information.

Save your search on a floppy disc before logging off so that you can come back to where you were if you want to continue to modify the search upon later reflection.

Appraise the evidence

Now that you have extracted the publications that seem most relevant to your own question from your search, the next steps are to decide how much reliance you can put on their contents and how far you can extrapolate from those papers to your own circumstances. This will involve deciding whether the studies described in the papers were well conducted or flawed, whether the population and setting studied were similar enough to your own circumstances for the results to be generalisable to your population or setting, whether sufficient people or things were studied for the results to be representative of larger numbers, and how you will weigh one paper against another if they report conflicting results or conclusions.

Critical appraisal is the assessment of evidence by systematically reviewing its relevance, validity and results to specific situations.

Critical appraisal:

► identifies the strengths and weaknesses of a research paper
► develops a better understanding of scientific principles and research methodology
► increases your capability to understand to what extent published literature is applicable to other circumstances.

The meaning of different research methods and terms

Bias

Systematic deviation of the results from the true values due to the way(s) in which the study was carried out.

Confidence interval

This describes the degree of confidence that can be placed on any statistical result. It describes the range of results from the subjects or things studied within which the investigator is 95% certain that the true population mean lies (the usual level of confidence chosen).

Confounder

A factor, other than the variables under study, which is not controlled for and which distorts the results, causing a spurious association.

Controlled trial

As for a randomised controlled trial (see relevant entry) without the randomisation element.

A controlled trial detects associations between an intervention and an outcome but does not rule out the possibility that the association was caused by an unrecognised third factor linking both the intervention and the outcome.

Controls

The subjects in a (randomised) controlled trial who are (randomly) allocated to receive either placebo, no treatment or the standard treatment.

Cost-benefit analysis (CBA)

Compares the incremental costs and benefits of a programme. Measures both costs and benefits in monetary values and calculates net monetary gains or losses (presented as a cost-benefit ratio).

Cost-effectiveness analysis (CEA)

Compares the effectiveness of two interventions with the same treatment objectives. Competing interventions are compared in terms of costs per unit of consequence. Consequences may vary but are measured in monetary terms.

Cost-minimisation analysis (CMA)

Compares the costs of alternative treatments that have identical outcomes.

Cost-utility analysis (CUA)

Measures the effects of alternative interventions in terms of a combination of life expectancy and quality of life, using utility measures such as quality-adjusted life years (QALYs), and may present relative costs per QALY.

Effectiveness

The extent to which an intervention does what it is intended to do for a defined population.

Efficacy

The extent to which an intervention produces a beneficial result under ideal conditions. Preferably based on an RCT.

Hawthorne effect

The influence of knowledge of the study on behaviour. The effect of being in a study on the persons being studied.

Incidence

The numbers or proportion of new cases of a disease or condition occurring within a population over a given period of time.

Intention-to-treat analysis

This is a quantitative estimate of the benefit of a therapy (for instance, folic acid) in the population being studied, derived from comparing control and treatment groups.

Meta-analysis

This is a method of combining two or more studies to obtain information about larger numbers of subjects. Inclusion criteria should be clearly stated in the method to enable different studies to be considered together. It should appear reasonable to treat the sum of the different studies as one whole and that like is being combined with like.

Number needed to treat (NNT)

A measure of the effectiveness of treatment. It tells you the number of people you would need to treat with an intervention over a given period of time to get one additional beneficial outcome or to prevent an additional adverse outcome.

Observational study

There are several types of study where the subjects are observed over time and the experiences are recorded or reported.

A cohort study is one where two similar groups of people who do not have the disease or condition under study are observed prospectively over a predetermined period to see the effects of one group being exposed to an already established suspected risk factor (such as cigarette smoking) and the other group not being so exposed.

A cross-sectional survey gathers information about subjects or things in a study population at one point in time or over a relatively short period.

Odds ratio (OR)

A measure of treatment effectiveness. The probability of an event happening as opposed to it not happening. An OR of 1 means that the effects of treatment are no different from no treatment. If the OR is greater than (or less than) 1, it means that the effects of treatment are more (or less) than those of the control group.

Placebo

An inert substance that is given to control subjects in trials.

Power

Sample sizes should be calculated before the study design is finalised, to determine the numbers needed for the study to be likely to detect a sufficient effect from the intervention, so as to be sure that the effect did not occur by chance alone. The power calculation predicts the number needing to be studied to detect an effect at least at the level of 95% significance. This is the level of certainty that is equal to or less than a one in 20 risk that the effect occurred by chance and was not due to an intervention or event being studied.

Prevalence

The proportion of 'cases' within a specified population at a given time.

Probability

Probabilities are often written as p values in published reports, where p stands for probability. It is a measure of how likely an outcome is. This lies between 0 (where an event will never happen) and 1.0 (where it will definitely occur).

The p value is a guide to whether the outcome measured occurred by chance or was due to the intervention or event that the study was designed to measure.

A significant p value is one where the likelihood is that the effect or outcome occurred as a result of the intervention or event being studied, and did not occur by chance. The most common convention is to decide arbitrarily on a one in 20 risk of being wrong about the direct causal relationship between the intervention or event and the outcome; that is, the risk that the outcome occurred by chance. This can be described as '$p = 0.05$', 'at the 5% significance level' or as a '5 in 100 probability' that the outcome occurred by chance. If written as '$p < 0.05$' there is less than 5 in 100 risk of the outcome having happened by chance. Smaller p values give increased confidence in the test results; for example $p < 0.001$ indicates that the probability that the outcome occurred by chance is less than one in a thousand. The level of significance the investigators choose should depend on the importance of being right about the intervention/outcome relationship, and the numbers in the populations being studied.

Sometimes investigators get carried away, testing every bit of data in their study to see if they can dredge up some significant results. This is very bad practice because even a short questionnaire can yield hundreds of combinations of possibilities if each question has several alternative categories of answers: for example, age might be subdivided into nine decades. If a significance test was applied to all the possible combinations of answers looking for potential links and 200 tests of significance were tried, for example, you would expect ten tests erroneously to indicate statistical significance where the outcome(s) had occurred by chance (that is, 5 in 100 risk $\times 2 = 10$). So the arbitrary $p < 0.05$ test of assumed significance is not cut-and-dried proof that an outcome is directly attributable to an intervention – it is just a good indicator of significance.

Publication bias

Results are more likely to be published if the results are positive rather than negative. Thus, it may appear that treatments have more positive results than is actually the case.

Randomised controlled trial (RCT)

Randomisation is necessary to minimise and, hopefully, eliminate selection bias. This is the type of study design which is most likely to give you a true result, because not all of the subjects or things in the trial are exposed to the intervention or factor being studied. The subjects or things are randomly allocated either to the group exposed to the intervention or to the control group who are not intentionally exposed to that intervention. The experiences and outcomes of both groups are compared to see if they are significantly different according to statistical tests. Sometimes the design includes more than two comparative groups.

Using the randomised controlled trial method distributes unsuspected biological variables equally between the two groups, as well as any other external factors of which you are unaware. Both the subject and control groups will be exposed to these unrecognised external influences (called confounding factors) and any differences in outcomes between the two groups should be attributable to the intervention being studied.

When the term 'randomised' is stated, there should be some information in the method as to how this randomisation process was carried out to minimise any external influences from interfering with the random allocation of subjects or things to different arms of the study.

If a trial is 'double blind', neither the clinician/investigator making the intervention or analysing the results, nor the person receiving the intervention, should know whether they are in the intervention or the control group. In a 'single blind' study, either the clinician or the subject knows to which group the subject belongs.

Relative risk

Relative risk is calculated by taking the ratio between two measures of risk. If there is no difference between two groups, the risk ratio is '1' as the risks in each group are the same. A risk ratio greater than '1' shows the outcome in the study group to be better than that for controls.

The risk ratio is the proportion of the group at risk in one group divided by the proportion at risk in a second group. The risk ratio is a measure of relative risk.

Reliability

A reliable method is one which produces repeatable results.

Sensitivity analysis

Tests the robustness of the results of an economic analysis by varying the underlying assumptions around which there is uncertainty.

Sensitivity of test

The true positive rate of a diagnostic test, that is, how often the test misses people with the disease.

Specificity of test

The true negative rate of a diagnostic test, that is, how often the test indicates people as having the disease when they do not.

Statistically significant

By convention taken to be at the 5% level ($p < 0.05$). This means that the observed result would occur by chance in only one in 20 cases (*see* Probability).

Systematic review

Systematic reviews of randomised controlled trials provide the highest level of evidence of the effectiveness of preventative, therapeutic and rehabilitatory treatments (as described in the section on hierarchy of evidence, pp 44–5).

Validity

A valid method is one which measures what it sets out to measure.

Reading a paper

Reading and evaluating a paper is mainly about applying common sense. Traditionally, critical appraisal of the literature has been made to seem like a difficult science for the elite, rather than a basic skill that any health professional can readily learn and apply to their own situation.

If you read a report of a research study and apply to it the questions on the page opposite, you will soon discover for yourself some of the common flaws in published studies, sometimes even those in respected peer-reviewed journals where the mistakes were not noted by the researchers or publication team.

In general you should consider whether:

- ▶ the paper is relevant to your own practice
- ▶ the research question is well defined
- ▶ any definitions are unambiguous
- ▶ the aim(s) and/or objective(s) of the study are clearly stated
- ▶ the design and methodology are appropriate for the aim(s) of the study
- ▶ the measuring instruments seem to be reliable; that is, different observers at different points in time would arrive at the same outcome

- ▶ the measuring instruments seem to be valid; that is, the investigator is actually measuring that which she/he intends to measure
- ▶ the sampling method is clear
- ▶ the results relate to the aim(s) and objective(s) of the study
- ▶ the results seem to be robust and justifiable
- ▶ the results can be generalised to your own circumstances
- ▶ there are any biases in the method of the study
- ▶ there are biases in the results, such as non-reporting of drop-outs from the study
- ▶ the conclusion is valid
- ▶ you have any other concerns about the study.

Specifically you should look at:

- ▶ where the study was done and who the authors are
- ▶ the study design: how were the subjects and controls selected, were they randomised and if so how, what were the outcome measures, were the outcome measures clinically relevant, are the sample numbers appropriate?
- ▶ the results: are the numbers of drop-outs and non-respondents reported, are all subjects accounted for, is the statistical analysis explained, are the results clearly presented?
- ▶ the discussion and conclusions: does the report describe the study's limitations, are the conclusions supported by the results?

Critical appraisal of a published paper or report of a study

1 The aim(s) and /or objective(s) of the study should be stated clearly.

   - ▶ The aim should state the purpose of the study succinctly and specifically. It should be set in the context of information that is already known from previously published literature.

▶ The reasons for, and need to carry out, the study should be justified in the introduction of the paper.

▶ There should be a clear route built up from the aim to the conclusion, flowing from the explanation of why a particular study design, population and setting were selected, to the results reported, the discussion and interpretation and final conclusion(s).

2 The methodology should be appropriate for the aim of the study.

▶ Quantitative and qualitative design techniques are complementary. A good quantitative survey will be based on prior qualitative work to determine what are appropriate questions to ask in the questionnaire or interview schedule. A randomised controlled trial may be a gold standard quantitative study design, but a qualitative method will most probably be needed to report people's observations, reflections and judgements.

▶ As a generalisation, prospective recording is more likely to be accurate than retrospective recall.

▶ A sample of a population should be selected for study which is as representative as possible of the whole population.

▶ A setting should be chosen for a study which is as representative as possible of the setting of the total population to which the results of the study will be extrapolated.

▶ The sample size should be justified by a *power calculation* determined prior to starting the study and based on the expected findings.

▶ There should be a method for increasing the response rate to as near as possible an ideal of 100% of the subjects included in the study.

▶ Details of any measurement or intervention should be as specific as possible, and transparently valid and reliable.

▶ A good study design will include a method to validate the questionnaire, rating scale or results obtained.

▶ It is always a bonus to see an original questionnaire even if only in an abbreviated form, to be able to judge for yourself the validity of the questions used in the study.

▶ The statistical methods should be described so that when the results are reported readers can check the statistical calculations and understand how the results were derived from the original data, if they wish.

3 The results should be robust, justified and related to the objectives of the study.

▶ The results should be simple to understand. It should be obvious where the results have come from and they should not seem to have been plucked out of thin air. Graphs and tables help to avoid strings of numbers and percentages.

▶ Statistically significant results should be presented in a conventional way or explained with full references if less well known statistical tests are used.

▶ Percentages should add up to 100%, and if they do not there should be some explanation to account for the missing numbers. It should be clear where and whether subjects have not sent back the questionnaire, have left a particular question blank or given a 'don't know' response.

▶ If the results obtained from the subjects are fairly crude, such as when people are asked to estimate their answers or recall happenings in the distant past, the result should be given as whole numbers or to one decimal place, rather than given as several decimal places which might look more scientific to the casual reader.

▶ The written contents of a research paper should be in their correct places. Bits of method should not crop up afresh in the results, nor should discussion be interspersed with the results. The flow of the paper should be logical and build up to a justifiable conclusion. Anything otherwise is confusion and muddle.

▶ A low response rate may mean that the results from the sample of the population studied are not likely to be representative of the whole population. The further you regress from a 100% response rate, the more likely it is that you have missed people or things that would give your results a different slant. As a very rough guide, a response rate of 70% seems generally to be regarded as reasonable for a topic where the results are not going to have dire consequences if they are wrong. But if the study was a trial of drug therapy where people's lives might be at stake if the research results and conclusions were wrong, anything less than a 100% response rate might be unacceptable.

4 Any biases in the design and execution of the study should be minimised and their likely influences acknowledged and explained.

▶ Good response rates are important because responders may have different characteristics from those of non-responders.
▶ There may be confounding factors present. These are so-far undetected influences that were not measured or recorded in the course of the study, but that were actually wholly or partly responsible for causing the changes or results reported. There are often cultural changes with time outside the study and beyond the control of those undertaking the investigation. For instance, if a famous celebrity claimed benefits for a new treatment that was being studied, many more people would suddenly believe they had received the same benefits and the outcomes being studied at that time would be distorted. Opting for *randomised controlled trials* avoids the influence of confounding factors.
▶ The potential and actual biases of the study should be openly described and their likely effects discussed in the Discussion section of the paper. Readers should then be able to make up their own minds about the relative importance of each bias on the results and how much

the biases prejudice the extrapolation of the results to the readers' own situations.

5 Is the conclusion valid?

► The conclusion is often found in the Discussion section of a paper when there is no separate Conclusion section.

► The conclusions of the results should not hinge on probability test results. The significance of the results claimed should make sense from clinical and common sense perspectives too. For example, an intervention might claim that it is significantly better than another at increasing small children's height by 0.1 inches. But if, clinically, this difference is inconsequential, then the benefits of the treatment claiming to be superior are not proven by the positive significant result.

► The conclusion(s) should not make any claims that have not been justified previously in the report of the study.

► No new information should suddenly crop up in the conclusions that was not previously cited in the method, results or another section.

► It should be clear what the main findings mean and what the implications are for current practice or future developments.

► The results of the current study should be compared and contrasted with others reported elsewhere and any discrepancies interpreted and discussed.

6 Any other concerns about the study.

► Conflicts of interest should be stated, such as the sponsorship of the study by a manufacturer of the medication tested in the study.

► Look for any omissions in any section of the report. Think whether the implications from any contrary results seem to have been considered in full or glossed over.

Examples

Critically appraise this example – a summary report of a research study.

1 An investigation of the use of sunscreens in the United Kingdom

Summary

Aim: To investigate the use of sunscreens in children.

Method: A postal questionnaire was sent out to all 942 members of Women's Institutes throughout the Scottish Isles, asking them about the frequency of the use of high-factor sunscreens applied to their children (please contact the author for a copy of the questionnaire). Questionnaires were anonymous to ensure confidentiality. An article was placed in the Women's Institute newsletter to prompt non-responders.

Results: 356 women replied (85% response rate; average age 56 + SD 16.4298 years). 290 stated that they bought factor 10 or higher sunscreen. 89 preferred the scent-free version ($p < 0.1$). 350 women thought that the Government should subsidise the cost of sunscreens as they were too expensive ($p < 0.0001$). The presence of a melanoma should be treated as a criminal offence and the sufferer fined for not having used sufficient sunscreen, as a contribution to the costs of the ensuing NHS treatment.

Conclusion: If the Government were to subsidise the cost of buying high-factor sunscreens, uptake would be increased and the frequency of melanomas or other skin cancers would fall.

Source of funding: Nibblea Suncreams.

Conflict of interest: None.

Chambers R (2001) *J Evidence-Based Spoof.* **3**: 12.

Consider the following challenges

Write down your answers then read the author's opinion below:

1 Are the aim(s) and/or objective(s) of the study clearly stated?

2 Is the methodology appropriate for the aim(s) of the study?

3 Do the results relate to the aims(s) and/or objective(s) of the study? Are the results robust and justified?

4 Are there any biases in the design and execution of the study?

5 Is the conclusion valid?

6 Are there any other concerns about the study?

Critique of the summary report: use of sunscreens in the United Kingdom

1 Are the aim(s) and/or objective(s) of the study clearly stated?

The aim is not very specific. If the focuses of the conclusion on cost of sunscreens and the impact of sunscreens on the frequency of cancers were intended as the purpose of the study, then the aim has been expressed incorrectly.

2 Is the methodology appropriate for the aim(s) of the study?

No, no, no! There is already confusion as the aim and conclusions are so far apart, but working on the premise of the aim stated in the summary of the study given:

▶ the population chosen for study is inappropriate as children of Women's Institute members probably range in age from 1 to 60 years old; this can be deduced from the subject's average age being 56 years and the standard deviation (SD) 16.4 years, indicating that about two-thirds of the population studied are between 40 and 70 years (that is, 56 − 16.4 years = 40 years to 56 + 16.4 years = 70 years)

▶ the Scottish Isles setting is in a part of the United Kingdom that would be expected to have relatively low amounts and strength of ultraviolet rays, and results from this setting cannot necessarily be generalised elsewhere

▶ members of Women's Institutes living in the Scottish Isles whilst the study was in progress had not necessarily lived there all their lives; so if the geographical area was important, the mothers do not have uniform histories of where they lived when younger, and their children may have lived apart from their mothers at any time previously

▶ the differing age range of the children means that some mothers' reports will relate to children under the age of 18 years currently receiving modern types of high-factor sunscreens, and others will relate to middle-aged children who may or may not have had old-fashioned creams applied a varying number of years previously; high-factor sunscreens did not exist at the time the study began

▶ there is no logic in choosing Women's Institute members as the population group to be studied – it may introduce a further bias if it were shown that members were more likely to be part of a more affluent section of society than the general population as a whole and therefore more likely to take holidays abroad where the sunshine was more powerful and potentially damaging

▶ mothers' recall of the frequency of use of suncreams applied to children up to 50 years before is unlikely to be accurate

▶ anonymous questionnaires that do not bear a code number make chasing up of individual non-respondents impossible – an article placed in a newsletter is unlikely to be an effective method of encouraging non-responders to reply.

3 Do the results relate to the aim(s) and/or objective(s) of the study? Are the results robust and justified?

It is obvious that the results are inaccurate and meaningless. Also:

- ▶ the response rate was very low at 38% (356/942), not 85% as stated
- ▶ the results, such as the information about costs of sunscreens, are not related to the data that would have arisen from the study method described
- ▶ it is ridiculous to give the standard deviation (SD) to four decimal places when the average age is given as a whole number
- ▶ a probability of <0.1 is not significant and no such conclusions can be drawn about a proportion of the population studied preferring the scent-free version
- ▶ results should be factual and not offer interpretations, as here where the Government is encouraged to treat the presence of melanomas as a criminal offence
- ▶ the results cannot be generalised.

4 Are there any biases in the design and execution of the study?

The study is riddled with biases from start to finish. Many have been described already, such as:

- ▶ the nature of the population
- ▶ that retrospective recall of information is likely to be poor
- ▶ the poor response rate
- ▶ the changing nature of commercially available sunscreens over time throughout the study
- ▶ the fact that the conclusion does not relate to the rest of the study, which implies that the whole purpose of the study may have been to prove that sunscreens should be subsidised and that the design and reporting of the study might be biased to that end.

5 Is the conclusion valid?

No it is not. It does not follow from the rest of the report and is not related to the original aim.

6 Are there are any other concerns about the study?

Although the author of this report states that there was no conflict of interest, the sponsorship of the study by a manufacturer of suncreams should alert readers to scrutinise the report even more carefully than usual for possible biases.

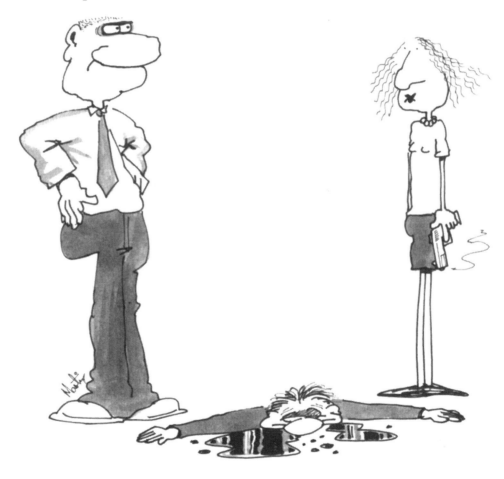

▼

Remember that sometimes the evidence can be misleading.

Critically appraise this second example – an unpublished report of a research study. Answer the following challenges, as before – write down your answers then read the author's opinion:

1 Are the aim(s) and/or objective(s) of the study clearly stated?

2 Is the methodology appropriate for the aim(s) of the study?

3 Do the results relate to the aims(s) and/or objective(s) of the study? Are the results robust and justified?

4 Are there any biases in the design and execution of the study?

5 Is the conclusion valid?

6 Are there any other concerns about the study?

2 Why do teenagers become pregnant?

The following report concerns a real study carried out by one of the authors (RC) but it has been much adulterated to illustrate the learning points. All of the faults described below frequently appear in published papers, although not usually to such an exaggerated extent. The subsequent critique picks out main points and is not intended to be comprehensive – you will note more errors and poor research practice.

Introduction: Nine out of 10 teenage mothers in one survey reported that their pregnancies were unplanned (Francome and Walsh, 1995). Most of these had not used contraception because sexual intercourse had been 'unexpected'. The younger the girl at first intercourse, the sooner intercourse had occurred in the relationship in one study of pregnant teenagers (Curtis *et al.*, 1988). Many had not sought formal advice about contraception from either family planning clinics or general practitioners because they thought it was illegal for those under 16 years of age to obtain contraceptives or that their parents must be told, or because they felt embarrassed. Pearson *et al.* (1995) reported that three-fifths of a cohort of pregnant teenagers had used condoms which had apparently leaked, split or come off.

About a fifth of women aged 16 to 49 years in England who require contraception go to family planning clinics and most of the rest go to general practitioners (Government Statistical Service, 2000). The proportion of teenagers aged under 16 years who visit family planning clinics for contraception has increased over the last 20 years and it is estimated that in 1999–2000 about 43 000 females aged 15 years attended (about 14% of the population aged 15 years), and 25 000 girls aged under 15 years (about 4% of the population aged 13 to 14 years old). The proportion of women aged 16 to 19 years old who attended family planning clinics in 1999–2000 was 23%.

This study set out to determine the reasons why teenagers became pregnant in one county in the Midlands of England.

Method: A questionnaire was devised to enquire about the circumstances and reasons why teenagers became pregnant, their past use of contraceptives, their knowledge about contraceptives, possible exposure to HIV and other sexually transmitted diseases, and their smoking status. Teenagers were also asked if they had received advice about their future contraceptive needs.

Midwifery and ward staff working on the maternity and gynaecology wards of one general hospital administered questionnaires to teenage patients aged 19 years and under during a three-month period. The research nurse visited each ward every week to collect the completed questionnaires.

Data from the questionnaires was analysed using the statistical package SPSS.

Results: There were 113 live births to teenagers and 57 teenagers had a termination of pregnancy during the 12-week study period. Seventy-one of the 113 teenage in-patients completed questionnaires about the contraceptive services they had received whilst on the ward, and reasons why they had become pregnant. Seventeen of the 57 teenagers who had a termination of pregnancy completed questionnaires too; one other patient who had a termination refused to complete a questionnaire. Ward staff told the research nurse that they had been 'too busy' to remember to administer questionnaires to all teenagers in their care.

Seventeen subjects completed their questionnaires within one day of giving birth, 29 between one and two days and 25 more than two days after delivery. Those who had terminations responded before being discharged later the same day.

The most common reason, given by 34% of teenagers, for becoming pregnant was that no contraception had been used. A third had intended to become pregnant. Ten per cent had forgotten to take their contraceptive pills, one patient reported failure of emergency contraception pills taken correctly and two patients had become pregnant whilst taking antibiotics in addition to the contraceptive pill. The rest described using condoms which had burst during sexual intercourse.

Table 1: Reasons for becoming pregnant given by teenagers who have had a live birth or termination of pregnancy

Reasons for pregnancy	Teenagers who have had live birth or termination (n = 88)
Planned	24
Forgot to take oral contraceptive (o/c) pill	9
Condom burst	13
Condom slipped off	2
Failure of emergency contraception	2
Took antibiotics whilst on o/c pill	2
Multifactorial	1
Did not use contraception	30
No response	3

Table 2: Midwives' perceptions about extent of contraceptive help given

Extent of help given	Number of teenagers who had live birth or termination (n = 88)
'Learnt all they needed to know'	62
Patient's time for questions limited	21
Did not want contraceptive advice	2
Family planning leaflets given	74
No family planning leaflets given	3
Patient did not want family planning leaflets	6

There was a significant difference between the reasons given for becoming pregnant by those who had a live birth, and by those who had had a termination, in that those who had given birth were significantly more likely to have planned their pregnancy ($p < 0.0001$).

Discussion: This study involved a wide range of teenagers with different experiences – both those who had had a live birth and those who had had a termination; so results can be generalised to teenagers in general.

There was a perception gap between midwives and other hospital staff believing that contraceptive advice had been given whilst on the ward and teenage patients reporting that they had received it. It may be that improved procedures in the provision of contraceptive advice should be developed so that the advice given has more impact on these young patients.

Teenagers viewed both family planning clinics and general practitioners' surgeries as important providers of contraceptive services. Young persons' clinics were not well known to these subjects.

A substantial proportion of pregnant teenagers had not used any form of contraception. This was probably because they had been unable to obtain the right help at the right time.

Condom failures were commonly blamed for unplanned pregnancies, usually because they burst; this should be investigated further to find out if bursting is due to inadequate fitting techniques or poor manufacture.

Conclusions: Teenagers who have just had a termination are ideally placed to receive contraceptive advice as they are 'trapped' in their hospital bed and should be motivated by not wanting to have another termination in the future.

Condoms should be more durable and much stronger so that they do not burst as easily.

The midwives in this study were lazy in that they only administered questionnaires to just over half the teenage patients in this study.

Teenagers find family planning leaflets very useful for giving them advice about future contraceptive needs.

References for the paper:
Curtis HA, Lawrence CJ and Tripp JH (1988) Teenage sexual intercourse and pregnancy. *Arch Dis Child.* **63**: 373–9.

Francome C and Walsh J (1995) *Young Teenage Pregnancy.* Middlesex University and Family Planning Association, London.

Government Statistical Service (2000) *NHS Contraceptive Services, England: 1999–2000. Bulletin 2000/27.* National Health Service Executive, London.

Pearson VAH, Owen MR, Phillips DR *et al.* (1995) Pregnant teenagers' knowledge and use of emergency contraception. *BMJ.* **310**: 1644.

Critique of the report: Why do teenagers become pregnant?

1 Are the aim(s) and/or objective(s) of the study clearly stated?

Yes, the aim is stated at the end of the introduction, but the aim given was much narrower than some of the other issues covered in the study. The bulk of the material given in the introduction concerns teenagers' usage rates of family planning clinics and sources of contraceptive provision, rather than literature focused on reasons for teenagers becoming pregnant. In the method section, enquiry was made about sexually transmitted diseases; and in the results and discussion sections, midwives reported whether they had provided contraceptive advice whilst teenagers were in-patients. The aim and objectives should cover the scope of the study.

2 Is the methodology appropriate for the aim(s) of the study?

▶ Interviews might have been more appropriate than an administered questionnaire to ensure that the interviewees understood the questions and in order to elicit sensitive information.
▶ The questionnaire should include young people's perspectives of their concerns and issues; so the method might have involved preliminary work with young people to gather their views and compose the questionnaire using their language and including their issues and priorities.
▶ There was no power calculation or indication of whether 88 subjects was a valid number to study and likely to give a reliable result.
▶ There was no mention of ethical approval having been gained, or subjects giving informed consent before participating in the study.
▶ Those administering the questionnaire (midwives and other ward staff) did not appear to be sufficiently involved in the research process and thus they often 'forgot' to administer the questionnaire to teenage subjects. It may also be that different midwives and other staff did not administer the questionnaire in an impartial way and biased the responses; and that there was variability between midwives and other ward staff in the way that questionnaires were administered.
▶ Subjects responded at varying times after delivery or termination, and this may have given them unequal opportunities for having received contraceptive advice whilst on the ward.

3 Do the results relate to the aim(s) and objective(s) of the study? Are the results robust and justified?

► The results from teenagers who had given birth, and those who had had a termination, should not have been added together as a joint result, without much more detailed analysis to check if the characteristics of both groups were so similar that adding their results together was justified. In this case, it seems the two groups of teenagers are very different and should be considered separately.

► There is an error in the figures in Table 1, which do not add up to the number of subjects (n = 88).

► There is a reference to SPSS but no mention of what statistical test was used to calculate the probability result.

► In Table 2 it is not clear if there were any non-respondents, and readers cannot check for themselves as midwife respondents appear able to give more than one answer, although this is not clear.

► The reports of the reasons for becoming pregnant are a mixture of percentages and actual numbers, so the actual results are omitted.

► There is too little information about the non-respondents and the reasons for non-response.

► As noted before, results are given that are outside the scope of the given aim. Some results are given for which there was nothing in the method section about how that information was collected, e.g. about midwives being asked for their perceptions of the extent of contraceptive help provided to teenage in-patients. Some information was described as being collected in the method (e.g. about sexually transmitted diseases), but for which no results are given. Some information is given in the discussion (e.g reference to teenagers' views about contraceptive help received) which does not appear in the results section.

4 Are there any biases in the design and execution of the study?

► The focus of the introduction on usage of family planning clinics and accidents with condoms, to the exclusion of literature reporting other reasons for teenagers becoming pregnant, seems to reflect a bias running through the whole study.

▶ There is not enough information about the subjects to understand if they are representative of teenagers in general. The study is confined to one general hospital somewhere in England and may not be generalisable to the general population of teenagers in the rest of England and beyond. So the method might have included comparison between different geographic locations, or collected more data about the socio-economic characteristics or educational attainment, etc. of subjects.

▶ The midwives and other ward staff who administered the questionnaires might have influenced the teenagers' completion of the questionnaires if they did not value the study and made known their feelings that it was a waste of time, or if the youngsters thought that the individual midwives would see their answers and they were reluctant to displease them.

▶ The timing of the study might have meant that the recent emotional and physical experiences of a live birth or termination affected the answers given by the teenage respondents.

5 Are the conclusions valid?

▶ Many of the conclusions are not justified by the results obtained. For instance, although 'burst' condoms were commonly reported, that may have been an excuse teenagers used rather than admit they had neglected to use contraception in the heat of the moment, or poor technique might have been the real reason for condoms failing. Extrapolating from the results to recommend that condoms be manufactured to be more durable is not supported by the findings of the study.

▶ The conclusion that immediately after a termination is an ideal time to provide contraceptive help, seems to have originated from the beliefs and preferences of the author of the study rather than information gathered during the research process.

▶ No information was gathered as to the workload of midwives on the wards. The supposition that they were 'lazy' because they did not prioritise administering questionnaires from the study in their everyday practice is a subjective conclusion of the author of the study that was not tested for, nor is it borne out by the findings.

▶ Teenagers were not questioned about how useful they found the information in the family planning leaflets they were given, according to the method that is described. It cannot be concluded that just because they received contraceptive literature they found it useful.

6 Are there any other concerns about the study?

▶ The question posed 'Why do teenagers become pregnant?' is a very widely-based question that will have a multi-factorial answer and cannot be answered in a healthcare setting alone – it should include social, educational and parenting elements at least.

▶ The timing does not seem appropriate for obtaining reliable and valid information to answer this question, coming as it does immediately after emotionally traumatic events such as giving birth or having a termination.

▶ There is no mention of consumer involvement in the form of teenagers themselves, in planning, undertaking or interpreting the results of this study.

Now critically appraise the report of a study you have identified from your search

1 Are the aim(s) and/or objective(s) of the study clearly stated?

2 Is the design appropriate for fulfilling the aims – the population, the setting, the sampling technique, the type of study, the methods of measurement, avoidance of biases or confounding factors? Are all stages of the design described

such that you could repeat exactly the same study if you had a mind to do so?

3 Do the results relate to the aim(s) and/or objective(s) of the study? Are the results robust and justifiable? Can the results be generalised to your own circumstances? Are the results clear? Are there mistakes in the results?

4 Are there any biases in the design and execution of the study? Are they discussed in sufficient detail and are allowances made for their effects?

5 Are the conclusion(s) valid? What do they mean for your own practice?

6 Have you any other concerns about the study?

Critical appraisal of a qualitative research paper

Although qualitative research is not part of the hierarchy of evidence, it can provide a useful source of evidence. Qualitative research has been used extensively in midwifery. Indeed, many midwives searching for evidence in respect of their field may find that while no quantitative research has been undertaken, there may be a number of published qualitative studies. Thus, it is essential that you are able to make a judgement about the quality of these types of study as well. The following checklist and reminders about features you should consider is modified from Greenhalgh and Taylor (1997).[32]

1 Did the paper address an important clinical problem? Was the research question clearly formulated and defined?
There should be a clear statement about why the research was done and the research question that was addressed.

2 Is a qualitative approach the best method of answering this research question?

Qualitative research is useful for exploring beliefs, feelings and perceptions; for gaining a deeper understanding of an area; for exploring situations where little is known; for exploring sensitive issues; for gaining the 'whole picture'; and for allowing participants to speak for themselves. If this is what is being done, then a qualitative approach is almost certainly best. But think whether a quantitative approach, such as a randomised controlled trial (RCT) would have been more appropriate.

3 Is the setting/context for the research clear? How were the subjects selected? Is the sampling strategy described in detail? Is this strategy justified?

Qualitative research is about exploring the beliefs and gaining a deeper understanding of the experiences of a particular group of people or individuals. The sample is therefore selected in order to include people from these groups. That is, people are chosen because they are part of that group, rather than being chosen at random or to represent the 'average' view.

4 Have the researcher's perspective, beliefs, experiences and background been taken into account?

'Researcher' or 'observer' bias is important in qualitative research, as the interviewer's background, knowledge, experience, beliefs etc. may have an influence on the results of semi-structured interviews and focus groups. It is impossible to eliminate researcher bias, so the authors should address this problem by discussing the researcher's perspective and how this might have influenced the interpretation of the results.

5 What data collection methods were used and are these described in detail?

Rigorous reporting of methods in articles about qualitative research is particularly important, as each study is unique in design and analysis. The methods tell the 'story' that is needed to interpret the results. Hoddinott and Pill (1997)[33] suggest that you should ask the following questions:

▶ *are the researchers' roles and qualifications clear?*
▶ *are interviewer details given?*

▶ *is the paper explicit about how respondents were recruited, who recruited them and how the research was explained to them?*

▶ *is it explicit about whether the interviewer was known to the respondents and how they were introduced?*

▶ *is the interview setting clearly stated?*

▶ *were methodological issues about the influence of the interviewer on the data addressed?*

6 What methods were used to analyse the data? What quality control measures were implemented? Was an attempt made to test the validity of the results? Was an attempt made to test the reliability of the results?

There are various different methods of analysing qualitative data, e.g. content analysis and grounded theory. You should look for evidence that the researcher has analysed the data in a systematic way. Do the authors state that the data, e.g. transcripts, field notes or audio tapes, are available for independent review? The authors should have looked for cases which contradict the developing theories. The data should have been independently analysed by another researcher, or a second researcher should have repeated the analysis.

7 Are the results credible? Are the findings clinically important?

Use your common sense and ask 'Do the results seem sensible and believable? Will they matter in practice?' You should also look at whether the authors present sufficient original data, e.g. verbatim quotes, and whether these are indexed to subjects so that they could be traced back and checked.

8 What conclusions were made? Are the conclusions justified by the results?

In qualitative research the results and the discussion are not separate as in quantitative research, as the results are an interpretation of the data. You can look for evidence that the conclusions are 'grounded in evidence', i.e. that they flow from the findings, how compre-hensible the explanations are, how well the analysis explains why people behave in the way they do, and how well the explanation fits with what is already known.

9 Can the findings be transferred to other clinical settings?
Qualitative research is often criticised for only being applicable to the setting in which it was conducted. However, if true theoretical sampling rather than simply convenience sampling has been used, then the results are likely to be more transferable.

The checklist outlined above is not as all-encompassing or universally applicable as a checklist for critically appraising quantitative research, as qualitative research is 'by its very nature, non-standard, unconfined, and dependent on the subjective experience of both the researcher and the researched'.[32] This checklist sets some useful ground rules which may be enhanced by information given in other sources.[33-37]

Critically appraise a review

Now that you have learnt to critically appraise a research report, try your hand at appraising a review. Refer back to the explanations about randomised controlled trials, probability, confidence limits or other scientific terms described in the earlier text if necessary. The same rules apply for carrying out a survey of all research about a topic as for individual research papers. The specific question being addressed must be stated explicitly, the subject population (relevant research reports) identified and accessed, appropriate information obtained in an unbiased fashion (by using specific criteria to identify which research reports should, and should not, be included in the review) and the final conclusions should relate the evidence obtained from the reviewed research reports back to the primary survey question.

Look particularly for information in the review to reassure you of the following:

▶ The topic and purpose of the review should be specified.
▶ The search methods used to find evidence relating to the question should be stated. The review of the literature

should be comprehensive – reasonable efforts should have been made to identify and include relevant studies by consulting a range of databases and tracking down 'grey' material such as that in books, conference proceedings, consensus statements or annual reports.

▶ The studies included in the review should be relevant and appropriate to the main subject or issue being addressed.

▶ Only similar data should have been combined from different studies with similar subject characteristics, circumstances and methodologies. The methods used to combine the findings of the studies included in the review should be stated.

▶ There should be enough details about the subjects, populations, settings and other important factors for you to be able to decide whether the review's results and conclusions will be relevant to your particular circumstances.

▶ The criteria used to define whether or not a study was included in the overview should be stated clearly in the methods section. The researchers should have adhered to those explicit inclusion criteria, avoiding any bias in their method of selection.

▶ The results should be presented clearly in a scientific way. The results should be understandable, numbers in tables should add up, and it should be obvious how any analyses were derived.

▶ The authors should describe how the quality of the papers was assessed – how many people assessed each paper, whether they were blinded to other researchers' opinions, what criteria of quality were used, whether these were valid, reliable and reproducible, and whether assessors adhered to the criteria.

▶ The results should be relevant to the declared aim of the review.

▶ The results should be generalisable – the significance of different biases should be considered and their implications discussed. The author(s) should give a critical analysis of the scientific rigour of the studies in the review, with all interpretative remarks being justified.

▶ The results should be comprehensive. Negative as well as positive findings in the different studies should be described.

The range of confidence limits gives more information than a mere probability statistic.

▶ The conclusions should be based on an overview of the data and/or analyses of all the studies included in the review.

▶ The outcomes should indicate clearly any modifications that should be made to future healthcare practice based on the evidence presented in the review.

If you want to practise your critical appraisal skills, obtain a copy of the following review about back pain. We have chosen this example as midwives often have to advise pregnant women about their back pain and recommend ways of reducing or controlling the pain:

▶ Waddell G, Feder G and Lewis M (1997) Systematic reviews of bed rest and advice to stay active for acute low back pain. *Br J Gen Pract.* **47**: 647–52.

Read through the article first to get a feel for it. Then read it again conscientiously absorbing the details and making notes as ideas and concerns come to mind. Now use the information given above, writing down your answers. The whole critical appraisal exercise should take you about three hours. Then read the section below and see how *we* reviewed this journal paper.

> **It may be hard to convince your colleagues even when you've got the evidence.**

Our review of Waddell *et al.* (1997)

This published review was prepared for the national *Guidelines on Acute Low Back Pain*,[38] an important and relevant problem in primary care. The following critique reflects the views of the authors and colleagues who attended the clinical effectiveness workshops. It is difficult to dissociate fact and interpretation in the critical appraisal of published papers and as several of the comments are matters of interpretation and opinion, you may well disagree with our critique.

Is the topic and purpose of the review clearly specified?

Yes. The aim was to review all randomised controlled trials of *bed rest* and of *advice to stay active* for acute back pain.

Were the search methods used comprehensive?

The search strategy was clearly stated and included searching Medline and Embase, hand searching and tracking down 'grey' materials. However, search of CINAHL was not included, which would have extended the search to include relevant literature from nursing and allied health disciplines, such as occupational therapy and physiotherapy.

Did the review address a clearly focused issue?

No. The inclusion criteria were too vague. For example, one of the inclusion criteria stipulated 'back pain of up to three months duration', but in some papers included in the review, the patients had had back pain for a few days, in others they had had pain for months. The inclusion criteria stated that trials of advice had to be set in 'primary care'. However, a very broad definition of primary care was used, e.g. three papers were set in occupational health clinics and emergency rooms.

The subjects in the bed rest studies and the advice populations were very different. That is, the settings, length of follow-up and outcome measures (most of which were irrelevant according to Table 3) were different, and, on the whole, smaller samples were used in the *bed rest* papers compared to those about trials of *advice*.

Some papers concerned primary care, while others concerned hospital outpatient care. They included studies of patients with recurrent attacks, acute exacerbation of chronic back pain and sciatica. These are all groups of patients for whom optimum care may well be different and some may benefit from bed rest whilst other groups may not. They should have focused on a particular group or groups of patients, symptoms or settings.

There was no discussion of outcomes and the difficulties in measuring them. To sum up a paper as showing that pain was 'worse' or 'better' ignores the difficulties in assessing pain over a period of weeks. The most severe pain experienced or the duration of pain above a certain level, the average pain score, pain at rest or pain on activity are all important features.

Did the authors look for the appropriate papers to include in the review?

No. They should have been more focused. For example, they could have identified a clinical question such as 'Should patients with acute onset back pain be advised to rest in bed until the pain subsides, or should they be encouraged to stay active?' Then they should have searched for papers that reported trials comparing these two alternatives. Instead they treated *bed rest* and *advice* to stay active as separate interventions and carried out two separate reviews.

Although the authors noted the problems with two of the papers and discussed them separately, they still included them in their review. For example, the paper by Pal *et al.* (1986) compared bed rest and continuous traction with bed rest and sham traction, which is a trial of traction and not a trial of bed rest at all. These papers should have been excluded.

The authors state in the method that back schools were excluded; however, one of the papers reviewed (Linequist *et al.*, 1984) is a trial of a back school.

Do you think the important, relevant papers were included?

No, papers on end-point evaluation have not been considered.

If the results of the review have been combined, was it reasonable to do so?

No, the studies have too little in common.

Did the authors do enough to assess the quality of the included studies?

No. There were too many dubious features of the scoring method used. The weighting of the criteria used for methodological scoring seems to have been accepted uncritically by the authors since it had been used in two other systematic reviews of back pain management. For example, an intention-to-treat analysis is one of the items (N) included in the methodological scoring system in Table 2. This is an essential feature, as a study loses nearly all of its credibility if it lacks this, and not just 5 points out of 100 as in the scoring system used by Waddell *et al*. 'Placebo controlled' is another one of the items (J) in the methodological scoring system. However, it is difficult to see how trials of bed rest and advice to stay active can be scored as to whether they are placebo controlled and how placebo bed rest might be arranged. A further problem with the methodological scoring is that the total sum in Table 2 is 100, yet the weightings given only add up to 95.

There is no substantive reason why co-interventions such as appropriate analgesia should be avoided in a study of back pain. To be realistic a trial protocol should allow appropriate analgesia, but should endeavour to ensure that patients in both groups are managed using the same guidelines with respect to analgesia. Use of analgesia could be an appropriate end-point to study.

What is the overall result of the review?

It is unclear because of the numerous flaws. The diversity of the studies in this area suggests that a more traditional type of review might be better, where papers are grouped under headings.

How precise are the results?

They only give results as 'better' or 'worse'. More precision is needed.

There are also several major mistakes. There is an inconsistency between Tables 2 and 3 in the total sum possible for the methodological scoring item F, which is given as 12 in Table 2 and 17 in Table 3. This accounts for the total adding up to 95 and not 100 as stated.

In Table 4 the asterisks and crosses in the last two entries appear to be mixed up. The asterisks should be crosses and the crosses should not be there.

Under *Methodological Quality*, the Spearman's rank correlation coefficient of 0.72 should not be interpreted as showing the rankings were similar – a value of 0.9 would be required.

The reporting of the results seems biased. In Tables 4 and 5 there are several instances where results are given as 'NS' (not significant) and several where the NS is elaborated on as 'slower recovery NS'. Where there is elaboration on NS, the detail, for example 'slower recovery (NS)', favours the final conclusion of the review. There must have been information available about all the 'NS' results and so the authors seem to have been selective in how much detail they present in order to favour their final conclusions.

Can the results be applied and generalised?

No, there are too many flaws. Furthermore, many of the studies included were not in primary care.

Were all important outcomes considered?

No, there is too little detail about outcomes, such as pain. Few of the important outcomes, such as time off work, were considered in the bed rest arm of the review.

Are the benefits worth the harms and costs?

This is unclear, given the flaws outlined above.

► STAGE 5

Apply the evidence

You have identified your problem, posed your question with help from colleagues at work, searched for the best available evidence, judged the quality of the evidence, weighed the relative importance of any conflicting results, applied the evidence theoretically to your own circumstances and situation, and now you should be ready to apply the evidence in practice.

Clinicians have expressed concern about the dangers of adhering blindly to evidence in practice, and fears that evidence-based practice might be regarded as the be-all and end-all as far as decisions about the cost-effective delivery of health services go. Clinical judgement and common sense must be paramount in keeping evidence in perspective. The information forming the 'evidence' may be irrelevant, incomplete or inaccurate, or the 'evidence' may simply not be applicable in the particular clinical circumstances in question. The NHS has a long way to go in accumulating a bank of good and reliable information about current clinical care and best practices.

Sir Douglas Black[39] warned about giving undue primacy to the evidence generated in randomised controlled trials. They may provide the best sort of evidence for evaluating the benefits of alternative medications, but they are not necessarily the best way of identifying evidence for resolving more complex human health issues.

Evidence-based management has an even weaker information base than evidence-based clinical practice. It must be right to encourage practice managers and other health service managers to adopt a research culture with a questioning approach. This will encourage them to reflect about what is happening, how and why, and to compare management practices.

So bear all this in mind as you think about applying the evidence you have gained from your search to your particular clinical situation. You may like to think of making changes from the perspective of an individual midwife, a team, maternity unit, or trust.

Diary of your progress in searching for evidence

Complete this summary of progress to date and your action plan for how you propose to introduce any changes in your working practices.

Write a summary of:

1 your problem (be as specific as possible so that you can measure the outcomes of any changes against this baseline position):

2 your question:

3 your search method – where you searched (databases, people):

4 the types of your best evidence (systematic review, randomised controlled trials, controlled trials, reports, conference proceedings, expert opinions):

5 give three titles of the most relevant and appropriate publications or sources that you found:

6 your conclusion(s) from the best evidence available in answer to your question:

7 the change(s) that you propose to make yourself or that others should make, as a result of the evidence you have obtained and the conclusion(s) you have drawn:

Action plan

People to whom you have fed back the results of the evidence.

Have you already written a timetabled action plan?   *Yes / No*

The baseline position:

Whom have you involved in discussions about the change(s) you propose?

Change(s) proposed:

People whom the proposed change(s) will affect:

Additional resources that will be required (people, premises, time, money, skills, etc.):

The timetable is:

Who will do what:

Advantages or health gains expected:

Disadvantages or losses (opportunistic costs) that may happen:

How and when the changed situation will be monitored again:

Barriers to change

Once evidence has been gathered, projects have been completed and necessary changes discussed, there can still be many barriers to overcome before worthwhile changes can happen.

The King's Fund PACE[6] initiative has identified the following barriers to change:

▶ others' lack of perception of the relevance of your proposed change (you should have realised this during your initial consultations with colleagues before you began)

▶ lack of resources to implement the change (time, staff, skills, equipment)

▶ short-term outlook of work colleagues

▶ conflicting priorities – without additional resources, changes have the potential to cause work overload or opportunity costs

▶ difficulties in measuring outcomes – it is difficult to find acceptable worthwhile health outcomes that are easily measured

▶ lack of necessary skills (forward planning is needed)

▶ no tradition of multidisciplinary working (this problem can probably only be surmounted with a culture change)

▶ limitations of research evidence on effectiveness (there's a lot more research about problems than there is about effective solutions)

▶ perverse incentives (a common flaw in the way the NHS functions)

▶ the intensity of others' contribution that is required (again consult early, get everyone on board and encourage everyone to 'own' your project).

And so ...

▶ anticipate the strength of evidence you will need to convince your colleagues that the efforts and costs of change will be worthwhile – to them and the clients. Do this through clinical governance – understand how to make clinical governance work for you in the next chapter.

Read more about the lessons to be learnt in how to make successful changes happen.[6]

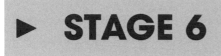

► **STAGE 6**

What clinical governance means and how to put it into practice

Clinical governance is inclusive, making quality everyone's business, whether they are a midwife or a doctor, manager or member of the administrative staff, a client or a strategic planner. We need to know where we are now and where we want to get to if we are to drive up standards of healthcare. Clinical effectiveness and clinical audit are central to this process.

Clinical governance 'is doing anything and everything required to maximise quality'.[40] It is about finding ways to 'implement care that works in an environment in which clinical effectiveness can flourish by establishing a facilitatory culture' where at the same time, underperformance is weeded out.[41–43]

Components of clinical governance

The components of clinical governance are not new. Bringing them together under the banner of clinical governance and introducing more explicit accountability for performance is a new style of working. The reception given to clinical governance has ranged from an enthusiastic welcome to the cautious warning that innovations that improve quality may increase rather than decrease costs. Carefully evaluating your work and demonstrating subsequent improvements in patient care will enable you to form your own view about the place of clinical governance.

The following 14 themes are core components of professional and service development which taken together form a comprehensive approach to providing high-quality healthcare services and clinical governance. These are illustrated in the tree diagram:[43]

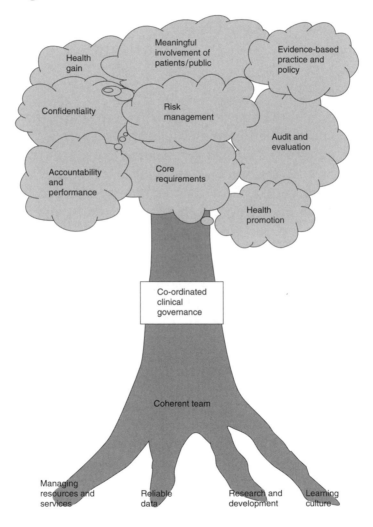

Figure 1   'Routes' and branches of clinical governance (© 2000 Chambers and Wakley)

If you interweave these into your individual and workplace-based personal and professional development plans, you will have addressed the requirements for clinical governance at the same time.[43]

1 **Learning culture**: in the maternity unit, the community, the trust and the NHS at large.
2 **Research and development culture**: throughout the health service.
3 **Reliable and accurate data**: in maternity services wherever they might be delivered and the NHS as a seamless whole.
4 **Well managed resources and services**: as individuals, as a unit or trust, across the NHS and in conjunction with social care and local authorities.
5 **Coherent team**: well integrated teams within a unit and across maternity services within a trust.
6 **Meaningful involvement of patients and the public**: in a unit or the NHS as a whole, including users, carers and the general population.
7 **Health gains**: activities to improve the health of patients in a unit, between hospital and community sectors and different geographical areas of the NHS.
8 **Confidentiality**: of information in consultations, in medical notes, between practitioners.
9 **Evidence-based practice and policy**: applying it in practice, in the trust, and across the NHS.
10 **Accountability and performance**: for standards, performance of individuals, the unit, the trust, health authority/board and the NHS, to the public and those in authority.
11 **Core requirements**: good fit with skill mix and whether individuals are competent to do their jobs, communication, workforce numbers, morale at practice level, across the NHS.
12 **Health promotion**: for patients, the public, opportunistic and in general, targeting those with most needs.

13 **Audit and evaluation**: for instance, of changes, of individuals' and units' performance, of the trust's achievements, of community services.
14 **Risk management**: pro-active review, follow-up, risk management, risk reduction.

The challenges to delivering clinical governance

Delivering high-quality healthcare, with guaranteed minimum standards of care for users at all times, is a major challenge. At present the quality of healthcare is patchy and variable. We aren't very good at detecting underperformance, and then taking the initiative and rectifying it at an early stage. The small number of clinicians who do underperform exert a disproportionately large effect on the public's confidence. Causes of underperformance in an individual might relate to a lack of knowledge or skills, poor attitudes or ill health. A lack of management capability is nearly always an important contributory factor to inadequate clinical services or the provision of healthcare.

We need to understand why variation exists and explore ways of reducing inequalities. Variation in the quality of healthcare provided is common – between different maternity units, between midwives working in the same practice or unit, between care given to some groups of the population rather than others.

Good practice means understanding and managing risk – both clinical and organisational aspects. Identifying new cases of important conditions such as gestational diabetes and undertaking audit more systematically will reduce the risks of omission – in detection and clinical management. The common areas of risk in providing healthcare services are thought to be:[44]

- ▶ out of date clinical practice
- ▶ lack of continuity of care
- ▶ poor communication

- ▶ mistakes in patient care
- ▶ patient complaints
- ▶ financial risk – insufficient resources
- ▶ reputation
- ▶ staff morale.

Clinical governance offers a co-ordinated approach to overcoming these areas of risk through the blend of clinical and organisational improvements to the quality of healthcare practice.

We need to agree on indicators of performance that are acceptable to clinicians and managers alike. It is often said that we tend to use outcomes that are the easiest to measure but which mean least in terms of the real quality of patient care.

Enhancing your personal and professional development

Education and training programmes should be relevant to service needs, whether at organisational or individual levels. Continuing professional development (CPD) programmes need to meet both the learning needs of individual health professionals and the wider service development needs of the NHS. You should no longer opt for CPD activities according to what you *want* to do, but rather, what you *need* to do. Clinical governance underpins professional and service development.[41]

Lifelong learning and CPD are integral to the concept of clinical governance and that includes everyone in a unit or team working towards agreed learning goals that are relevant to service development.

Good morale and job satisfaction are prerequisites of learning and effective working, and should be nurtured by targeted personal and professional development plans. Clinical governance should be creating a culture and working environment where people thrive and feel fulfilled by their work.

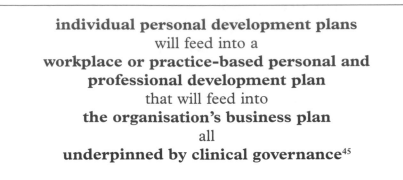

individual personal development plans
will feed into a
**workplace or practice-based personal and
professional development plan**
that will feed into
the organisation's business plan
all
underpinned by clinical governance[45]

The UKCC[18] introduced PREP to ensure that continuing professional development was recognised as a link between continuing education and practice development that resulted in improved standards of care. Clinical governance provides a framework for midwives to improve practice and facilitate clinical effectiveness, whilst fulfilling PREP requirements in a meaningful and satisfying way. This requires sustained CPD coupled with demonstrable high standards of care – clinical governance principles are integral to the process. The principles that underlie a review of the quality of the resulting service include:[46]

▶ the criteria for assessment of the quality of the service reflect the needs of patients
▶ professional self-regulation is the most effective and acceptable method of maintaining good professional practice
▶ the ethos should be educational, developmental and supportive
▶ every member of the team can take part
▶ the focus is the team, its functioning and the services it provides
▶ assessment of the quality of the service should be multi-disciplinary
▶ there should be local ownership and delivery.

1 How evidence-based care, clinical effectiveness and other components of clinical governance fit together: the practitioner's or the unit's perspective[43]

Learning culture

You cannot learn about the cultural changes needed for providing multidisciplinary, team-based healthcare in the modern health service by sitting passively in a lecture. You need to experience the learning and interact with others who will be part of that new culture. Historically, midwives have been keener to attend lectures than interactive educational activities such as organised small group sessions or informal teaching in their workplaces.

> The type or mode of education and training should be relevant to the topic of the learning and the characteristics or circumstances of the 'students'.

Maximising learning about the new requirements of the NHS will involve:

- ▶ setting up in-house formal and informal education and training opportunities
- ▶ everyone creating personal development plans that incorporate all modes of learning: reading and reflecting, shadowing others, small group discussions, online materials, as well as lectures and seminars
- ▶ a unit- or directorate-wide approach to a topic so that a portfolio of experience is built up to which everyone contributes – useful towards achieving PREP requirements.[18]

Applying research and development in practice

One of the most common research and development activities undertaken by health professionals is a questionnaire survey of their patients. A poorly designed patient satisfaction survey will give you meaningless results so that all the time and effort spent on the satisfaction survey is wasted, and changes made as a result of such a survey still will not satisfy the patient population. Patient satisfaction questionnaires are commonly used in hospital and general practice, as a hybrid of research and audit. Novices may mistakenly believe that undertaking a questionnaire survey is one of the simplest and easiest methods.

> Using a questionnaire is full of pitfalls and it is one of the most difficult techniques for gaining a true or valid answer to the question posed.

To try and ensure that a patient satisfaction survey is a meaningful exercise:

► use a questionnaire that has been tried and tested by someone else and is valid for your healthcare setting
► make sure that the questions are relevant and appropriate to the purpose of the enquiry
► use questions which have an easily answered format with simple choices of response
► use appropriate language likely to be understood by all respondents, with translations into other languages if there are non-English speakers in your target population
► avoid leading questions that imply you are expecting a particular answer, otherwise respondents will tend to give the answer implied as being the 'right' one because they want to please you
► pilot your draft questionnaire to detect problems with your questions or method.

Reliable and accurate data

Midwives, patients and administrators need reliable and accurate data to connect individuals or their healthcare records to other knowledge that is relevant to the care of the patient.[43]

Maternity services have led the way for other specialty services with shared and hand-held records between health professionals and patients. But it is generally health professionals who complete the hand-held record card, and more research is needed to explore the potential for both patients and health professionals to complete patient-held records.

Electronic patient-health records are becoming increasingly common and important for midwives. They can:

▶ record the information once
▶ record the information accurately by using templates or on-screen prompts
▶ display the information in a variety of ways, such as a summary, an episode, or a chronological account, or a stock list, a waiting list, a priority group for action
▶ make the information accessible by a variety of people from clinicians to administrators and policy makers
▶ make each part of the information subject to different levels of access so that, for example, personal medical information is not available to the accounts clerk
▶ supplement information not easily available by other means, such as how long people wait when they attend for their appointment
▶ be consulted remotely across long distances.

A paper record has inherent disadvantages: it cannot be in two places at once, it is difficult to find the information you want in a mass of paper sheets, it is inefficient – time is wasted looking for the record, looking in the record, copying out information that is in it – and it is bulky and difficult to store efficiently.

Make records easy to use so that you:

▶ minimise the training needed to use them

- prevent security procedures being circumvented
- record or retrieve information at the correct time
- reduce repetitive routine tasks
- enter or retrieve information in a standardised manner
- facilitate communication between all health staff
- incorporate audit and risk management
- base management and policy decisions on accurate information.

Well managed resources and services

The things you need to achieve best practice should be in the right place at the right time and working correctly every time. Systems should be designed to prevent and detect errors. So keep systems simple and sensible, and inform everyone how systems operate so that they are less likely to bypass the system or make errors.[43]

The objectives for clinical improvement for midwives may include:

- identifying problem areas and making recommendations to the midwifery lead
- assessing clinical risk and implementing corrective action
- communicating potential risks to patients, midwives and other support staff
- examining clinical incidents or complaints and recommending remedial action
- consulting the public about identifying service changes needed
- developing guidelines, standards, audit, procedures, care pathways, clinical policies and other actions to improve or change midwifery practice
- identifying training needs and making recommendations about implementation
- providing a forum among midwives for open discussion of performance monitoring, problems and development.

Coherent team work

Teams do produce better patient care than single practitioners operating in a fragmented way. Effective teams make the most of the different contributions of individual clinical disciplines in delivering patient care. The characteristics of effective teams are:

► shared ownership of a common purpose
► clear goals for the contributions each discipline makes
► open communication between team members
► opportunities offered for team members to enhance their skills.

A team approach helps different team members adopt an evidence-based approach to patient care, by having to justify their approach to the rest of the team.[47]

There can be professional hostility between NHS-employed and independent midwives, and this can be confusing for patients served by both. A cohesive team will find ways of overcoming such hostility and working together for the good of the individual patient.

Meaningful involvement of patients and the public

The terms 'user' and 'public' are employed here to include patients or users, carers, non-users of services, the local community, a particular sub-group of the population and the general public.

If user involvement and public participation is done well, it should result in:

► reductions in health inequalities
► better outcomes of individual care
► better health for the population
► better quality and more locally responsive services
► greater ownership of health services
► a better understanding of why and how local services need to be changed and developed.

Public participation may be organised at five levels, and you should aim for true participation at the fifth level whenever possible:[48]

- ▶ **Level 1**: information exchange
- ▶ **Level 2**: consultation: the public and patients express their views but the consultant makes the decisions
- ▶ **Level 3**: support: the public decides what to do and others support them in doing it
- ▶ **Level 4**: deciding together: thinking and planning together
- ▶ **Level 5**: acting together: putting plans into action together.

A meaningful public consultation involves the exchange of information between the healthcare providers and the general public, obtaining a representative opinion as a result that feeds into the local decision-making process of healthcare services or whoever is sponsoring the consultation.

How to go about undertaking meaningful consultation[49]

Be clear about:

- ▶ the purpose of the exercise: is it important and is it necessary?
- ▶ the type and identity of the population to whom the purpose relates
- ▶ how to reach and engage the target population
- ▶ the extent and mode of information exchange required prior to consultation
- ▶ the implications of the methods you employ in the consultation – what outputs you expect from the consultation
- ▶ how you will act on the results of the consultation
- ▶ how you will feedback the outcome of the consultation exercise
- ▶ how you will evaluate the consultation exercise.

You may have to trade-off a relatively cheaper method of consultation that engages with fewer people or with a less representative section of the population sub-group; if you do, you will need to understand what biases are arising and make allowances for those biases when you interpret the results of the consultation.

Health gains

The two general approaches to improving health are the 'population' approach, focusing on measures to improve health through the community, and the 'high risk' approach, focusing on vulnerable individuals who are at a high risk of the condition or hazard. We adopt a population approach for promoting the taking of folic acid before conception, and stopping smoking. We target vulnerable groups, such as looked-after children and those who have left care, to promote safe sex.[43]

The two approaches are not mutually exclusive and often need to be combined with legislation and community action. Health goals include:

▶ a good quality of life
▶ avoiding premature death
▶ equal opportunities for health.

Modifiable risk factors with potential health gains for pregnant women to reduce the risks of adverse effects on their foetus, as well as to enhance their own health, include:

▶ obesity
▶ lack of exercise
▶ excessive alcohol intake
▶ smoking.

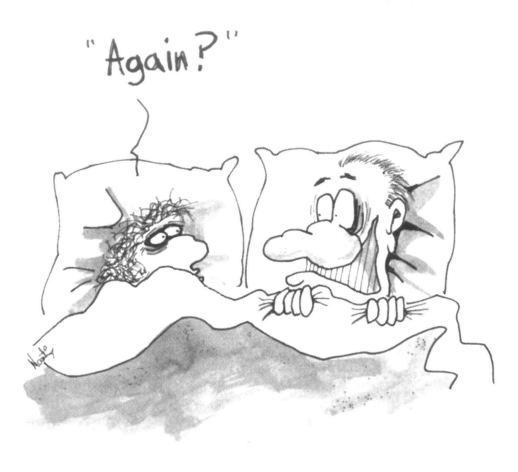

▼

Once you've tried to apply clinical effectiveness – you'll want to do it again!

Confidentiality

Confidentiality is a component of clinical governance that was often overlooked in the workshops which informed this book. Experienced midwives and managers may assume that junior or new staff know all about confidentiality but, of course, they may not. There are many tricky situations where one person asks for information about another's medical condition – test results or a progress report – where it is not clear cut as to whether this information should be supplied or withheld, or even if the person asked should acknowledge that the person enquired about is under their care. If the person in question is over the age of 16 years and has had a termination of pregnancy, then her medical attendants will not be able to share medical information without the patient's express permission, nor even indicate that she is receiving healthcare.

The Caldicott Committee Report[50] describes principles of good practice to safeguard confidentiality when information is being used for non-clinical purposes:

▶ justify the purpose
▶ do not use patient-identifiable information unless it is absolutely necessary
▶ use the minimum necessary patient-identifiable information
▶ access to patient-identifiable information should be on a strict need-to-know basis
▶ everyone with access to patient-identifiable information should be aware of his or her responsibilities.

Evidence-based culture: policy and practice

The key features of whether or not local guidelines worked in one initiative were that:[51]

▶ there was multidisciplinary involvement in drawing them up
▶ a well described systematic review of the literature underpinned the guidelines with graded recommendations for best practice linked to the evidence
▶ ownership was nurtured at a national and local level
▶ a local implementation plan ensured that all the practicalities (time, staff, education and training, resources) were foreseen and met, stakeholders were supported, predictors of sustainability addressed – guideline usability, individualising guidelines to practitioners and patients.

Clinicians may rebel against new policies that they perceive as being out of line with patients' needs, and policy makers may become frustrated at the intransigence of those in practice

– if there is a gulf between those driving policy and those responsible for practice. The evidence base justifying health policy and management decisions in relation to a particular service is just as important as the evidence base for the clinical care component of the service or the education of staff providing that service.

> Incorporating research-based evidence into everyday practice should promote policies on effective working and improve quality and a clinical governance culture.

▶ Be sure of the evidence for a proposed policy and the best way to implement it. Search for the evidence or set up a formal evaluation where there is insufficient evidence of the best way.
▶ Consult widely and early when any policy decision is being made, demonstrating how the input to that consultation was incorporated into the final policy.
▶ Base management and policy decisions on accurate information.
▶ Negotiate necessary changes in the organisation and management of practice and carefully cascade information about the changes throughout the unit or team or organisation.
▶ Provide adequate resources to underpin strategies to change practice, such as people to promote that change who have the right levels of knowledge and skills.
▶ Incorporate monitoring and evaluation of the change from the planning stage and throughout the activity.
▶ Find ways to maintain and reinforce the new practices, e.g. reminder systems, educational outreach programmes.
▶ Disseminate information about the change in ways that are appropriate to the nature and setting of the participants.

Accountability and performance

Statutory supervision of midwives is designed to 'safeguard and enhance the quality of care for the childbearing mother and her family'.[52] Supervision allows support for and review of practice for each individual practising midwife and, as such, contributes to clinical governance. The scope of midwifery accountability is set out in the Midwives Rules and the Code of Practice[53] and is discussed as part of supervision.

However, midwives may not always realise to whom they are accountable from outside their own profession. In fact they are accountable to:

▶ the general public – who are entitled to expect high standards of healthcare
▶ the midwifery profession – to maintain standards of knowledge and skills of the profession as a whole
▶ the Government and employers – who expect high standards of healthcare from the workforce.

Midwives who believe that they are not accountable to others may be reluctant to collect the evidence to demonstrate that they are fit to practise, and that their working environment is fit to practise from, the basis of the evidence for revalidation of their professional qualifications. In addition, they may not co-operate with central NHS requirements such as the National Service Frameworks.

Identify and rectify underperformance at an early stage by:

▶ regular appraisals (at least annually) linked into clinical governance and personal development plans. Appraisal is a process of regular meetings between manager and staff member with support for the benefit of the member of staff
▶ detecting those who have significant health problems and referring them for help

> ▸ systematic audit that detects individuals' performance as opposed to the overall performance of the midwifery team
> ▸ an open learning culture where team members are discouraged from covering up colleagues' inadequacies, so that problems can be resolved at an early stage.

Health promotion

People may under-estimate relative risks as applied to themselves and their own behaviour, e.g. many smokers accept the relationship between smoking tobacco and disease, but do not believe that they are personally at risk. People usually have a reasonable idea of the *relative risks* of various activities and behaviours, although their personal estimates of the *magnitude* of risks tend to be biased – small probabilities are often over-estimated and high probabilities are often under-estimated.[54]

> You need to understand the terms used to be able to extrapolate the messages from a research paper to explain the risks and benefits to others. You need critical appraisal skills to be able to form an opinion as to whether you can depend on the results from a research study.

Audit and evaluation

We should be looking for ways of assessing qualities like kindness, empathy, clinical reasoning and listening skills, as well as more tangible measures of the quality of care.

Clinicians may see the performance assessment framework as a management tool that is not particularly relevant to their clinical practice; this attitude will obstruct a coherent improvement programme if managers and clinicians have different goals.

> ▸ Communicate the meaning and implications of the performance assessment framework and indicators of achievement to individual units and practitioners.

▶ Incorporate the components of the framework into the maternity unit/trust-wide audits of practice performance, feeding back comparable data to individual units, teams and practitioners.

Analysis of critical incidents should focus on organisational factors as well as on the performance of particular individuals.

Core requirements

You cannot deliver clinical governance without well trained and competent staff, the right skill mix of staff and a safe and comfortable working environment, all providing cost-effective care.

Following published referral guidelines may increase health-care costs, which should be justifiable as cost-effective care when all direct and indirect costs are taken into account.

Your healthcare team can do much under the umbrella of clinical governance to respond to the national challenges to improve:

▶ partnership: working together across the NHS to ensure the best possible care
▶ performance: acting to review and deliver higher standards of healthcare
▶ the professions and wider workforce: breaking down barriers between different disciplines
▶ patient care: access, convenient services, empowerment to take a full part in decision making about their own medical care and in planning and providing health services in general
▶ prevention: promoting healthy living across all sections of society and tackling variations in care.

Risk management

Risk management in general practice or a trust mainly centres on 'facts' rather than 'values' or 'preferences'. These are the facts about what the probability is that a hazard will give rise to harm – how bad is the risk, how likely is the risk, when will the risk happen if ever and how certain are we of our estimates about the risks? This applies just as much whether the risk is an environmental or organisational risk in midwifery practice, or a clinical risk.[54]

Communicating and managing risks with individual patients is very much about finding ways to explain risks and elicit people's values and preferences, so that all these dimensions can be incorporated into the decisions they make themselves, to take risks or choose between alternatives that involve different risks and benefits.[54] A well functioning system through which patients can make complaints and receive feedback on the outcome should allow the practice or unit to reduce the risk of a recurrence.

2 How evidence-based care, clinical effectiveness and other components of clinical governance fit together: the maternity unit's or trust's perspective[43]

The 14 components of clinical governance described apply just as much to the approach required by a maternity unit as they do to teams and individual midwives. But the unit must also set up:

- clear lines of responsibility and accountability for the overall quality of clinical care in the unit[55]
- a systematic approach to monitoring and developing clinical standards in practice
- a comprehensive programme of quality improvement systems including workforce planning and development
- education and training plans
- clear policies aimed at managing risk
- integrated procedures for midwives to identify and remedy poor performance

▸ a culture where education, research and sharing good practice are valued.[56]

Clinical governance will be part of a culture of learning and the organisation will have an ethos of participation – for midwives and patients to engage in quality improvement.

The threats to a coherent clinical governance programme perceived by a group of practitioners at a local workshop were:

▸ lack of consensus about evidence-based practice and team-work
▸ lack of understanding of priorities
▸ 'What's the point if no resources for change?'
▸ 'blame' culture – way of thinking
▸ geographic isolation of some midwives and units
▸ lack of trust and information about skills between employed and independent midwives
▸ fear of new things/deficit in skills to cope with rapid change
▸ lack of time to fit new things in and get involved
▸ maternity units may find providing comparative data threatening
▸ clinical governance leads may be seen as 'know-it-alls' and 'do-it-alls' by other midwives
▸ few practitioners have personal development plans and many are unsure how best to proceed to blend clinical governance in with continuing professional development
▸ there is a lack of ownership of the importance of clinical governance by midwives
▸ clinical governance is seen as a threat and as a top-down imposition by some practitioners (not all)
▸ lack of multidisciplinary culture or ownership – not all members of the team see themselves with a part to play in clinical governance
▸ there are anxieties about how information on performance will be used and interpreted
▸ staff sickness levels may create variations in the delivery of services and blips of underperformance

- lack of systematic training
- the many initiatives may raise patient expectations above the capacity to deliver
- turnover of midwives in some units may be detrimental, e.g. loss of experience in implementing clinical governance
- lack of opportunities/willingness to learn about clinical governance in some units
- low level of public involvement, so standards are set by healthcare staff rather than the public
- units not all using the same IT hardware or recording systems, so peer audit is more difficult
- lack of co-ordination and updating of data about morbidity, consultations etc
- worries about identifying weaknesses as source of blame
- midwives may not see the wider context of the contributions of non-health organisations to improving health, nor understand each others' roles or the potential of the services each offers.

One review of how clinical governance was evolving in NHS trusts concluded that clinical governance could be simplified into five themes:[57]

1 policy emphasis on national consistency
2 accountability being at the heart of clinical governance
3 co-ordinating and linking audit, clinical effectiveness, complaints and risk management with an over-arching and coherent system of quality improvement and assurance
4 the assumption of responsibility for the management of poor performance and the promotion of clinical quality by chief executives leading to appraisal systems within trusts, external inspection, hospital doctors taking part in national audit
5 collaboration and teamwork between professionals.

One hospital's approach to clinical governance was to reform the senior committee structure to reflect:[58]

- leadership at different levels
- multidisciplinary style
- active co-ordination of the different elements of the committee, and of the hospital
- sharing of work across the service.

To achieve this, lead roles and responsibilities were allotted so that:

- evidence-based practice was led by a consultant
- risk management was led by a psychologist
- a nurse manager led on policy and procedure
- the senior occupational therapist led on clinical audit
- a general manager led on user issues and complaints.

3 How evidence-based care, clinical effectiveness and other components of clinical governance fit together: a district-wide perspective[43]

The district perspective is to take an overview, to check that national priorities are being satisfactorily translated into local prioritised action and that the anticipated outcomes of clinical governance are happening to reduce inequalities, and raise standards of healthcare in a uniform way across the district. The district perspective will be centred around the health improvement programme which should have been put together and actioned by all the NHS family and relevant non-health organisations.

Publishing information about achievements as league tables of professionals or organisations may worry patients and the public unnecessarily; and annoy health professionals who feel that any disadvantages about the context in which they work have not been fully taken into account. Highlighting any aspect of clinical governance may alarm the public in any case, if they think that any new initiative indicates that there is currently a lack of quality standards in place.

Clinical governance is a compulsory feature of all publicly funded healthcare services but not of the private sector (yet). This may cause tensions between the two if staff drain from one sector to another in response to different working conditions or financial incentives.

Clinical governance should be integral to any district strategies that promote high-quality healthcare. The strategy should encourage equity between primary care organisations and between trusts in the same district and a co-ordinated approach to quality improvement between the NHS and other organisations with an influence on health – education, local authority departments such as housing and police, voluntary organisations etc.

► EVALUATE YOUR NEWLY GAINED KNOWLEDGE AND SKILLS IN CLINICAL EFFECTIVENESS AND CLINICAL GOVERNANCE

Evaluate how much you have learned by doing this questionnaire and comparing your answers to questions 1 and 2 below with the equivalent questions in your initial self-assessment of your knowledge and skills about the topic at the beginning of this book.

Please circle as many answers as apply or fill in the information requested.

1 How confident do you feel *now* that you know enough about clinical effectiveness to be able to:

Ask a relevant question?	*Very*	*Somewhat*	*Not at all*
Undertake a search of the literature?	*Very*	*Somewhat*	*Not at all*
Find readily available evidence?	*Very*	*Somewhat*	*Not at all*
Weigh up available evidence?	*Very*	*Somewhat*	*Not at all*
Decide if changes in practice are warranted?	*Very*	*Somewhat*	*Not at all*
Make changes in practice as appropriate?	*Very*	*Somewhat*	*Not at all*

2 Which databases(s) have you used in your study?

CINAHL   Medline   Cochrane   Internet   Other (what?)

3 What level of evidence did you find in answer to your question (or main question if you posed more than one question)?

Strong evidence from at least one systematic review of multiple, well-designed randomised controlled trials (RCTs).

Strong evidence from at least one properly designed RCT of appropriate size.

Evidence from well-designed trials without randomisation.

Evidence from well-designed non-experimental studies from more than one centre or research group.

Opinions of well-respected authorities, based on clinical evidence, descriptive studies or reports of expert committees.

No evidence at all.

4 To whom have you given a report about the evidence you found?

Colleagues at work   Friends/family   Bosses (managers)   Other (who?)

5 What is/are the outcome(s) of your asking your main question and finding the evidence?

Made change(s) to an aspect of work – if so, please describe what change(s) you have made or plan to make, who was involved in deciding to make the change(s), who is involved in the new change(s), whether you need any more resources or training, and how you will review the change(s):

Decided against making any change(s) to any aspect of work – if so, why did you decide not to make any change(s) and who was involved in that decision?

Other outcome – what?

6 How will you use your new-found knowledge about clinical effectiveness in the future?

7 You have just been appointed as the clinical governance lead in your workplace. What are your roles and responsibilities likely to be and how will you go about promoting a positive culture of clinical governance among your team members?

Write down your answers – you can glean the information you need from Stage 6, which is the chapter on applying clinical governance in practice.

► USEFUL PUBLICATIONS OF EVIDENCE ALREADY AVAILABLE

Some evidence is already available, so it is not necessary to appraise all the evidence yourself. The following resources will be useful.

Bandolier is a UK newsletter published by the NHS Executive, Anglia and Oxford, which provides key evidence about the effectiveness of healthcare and keeps purchasers up-to-date with both local and national initiatives. It is free within the NHS in England and Wales. It is available in full text on the Internet at http://www.jr2.ox.ac.uk/Bandolier/. Non-NHS subscriptions are available from Hayward Medical Communications, Rosemary House, Lawades Park, Kentford, Newmarket, Suffolk, CB8 7PW. To register, email bandolier@pru.ox.ac.uk.

Clinical Evidence is a compendium of evidence on the effects of common clinical interventions, published by the BMJ Publishing Group. It is updated and expanded every six months and summarises the best available evidence about the prevention and treatment of a wide range of clinical conditions. Plus points are that its contents are driven by questions rather than by the availability of research evidence and so it identifies gaps in the evidence, leaving you to make your own decisions. Annual subscription costs £75 for individuals. However, an electronic version of Issue 4 is free on the Internet for NHS staff from work or with a password from home. For more details see http://www.evidence.org/ or http://www.nelh.nhs.uk.

Clinical Guidelines from the US Agency for Health Care Policy. Full text guidelines and summaries of the systematic reviews on which they are based. See http://text.nlm.nih.gov.

Drug & Therapeutics Bulletin provides independent evaluations of drugs and other medical treatments and management issues. It is available from the Consumers' Association, Castlemead, Gascoyne Way, Hertfordshire SG14 1LH or at http://www.which.net/health/dtb/cd.html.

Effective Healthcare Bulletin provides summaries of systematic reviews produced by the NHS Centre for Reviews and Dissemination and is designed to help NHS decision makers make more informed decisions by presenting the latest available information on the effectiveness of particular health service interventions. The bulletins are based on a systematic review and synthesis of the literature on clinical effectiveness, cost effectiveness and acceptability of health service interventions. It is available from the Subscriptions Department, Pearson Professional, PO Box 77, Fourth Avenue, Harlow CM19 5BQ or at the CRD website http://www.york.ac.uk/inst/crd.

Effectiveness Matters is produced by the NHS Centre for Reviews and Dissemination to complement *Effective Health-Care*. *Effectiveness Matters* provides updates on the effectiveness of important health interventions for practitioners and decision makers in the NHS. It covers topics in a shorter and more journalistic style, summarising the results of high-quality systematic reviews. Topics have relevance to primary healthcare. It is distributed free within the NHS – to subscribe, inform the Publications Office. The full texts of most of the *Effectiveness Matters* series can be viewed on the Internet at http://www.york.ac.uk/inst/crd or are available from the NHS Centre for Reviews and Dissemination, University of York, York YO1 5DD.

Evidence-Based Medicine provides critical appraisals of systematic reviews and primary research, with a commentary from a clinical expert. The journal is available on the *Best Evidence* database at http://hiru.hirunet.mcmaster.ca/ and from the BMJ Publishing Group, PO Box 299, London WC1H 9TD.

Guide to Clinical Preventative Services (2e). Evidence-based recommendations on preventive services. It is available at http://text.nlm.nih.gov/.

Journal of Clinical Effectiveness publishes papers on clinical effectiveness, evidence-based practice, guidelines and audit. Contact details: Financial Times Professional Ltd, PO Box 77, Subscriptions (Journals) Department, Harlow, Essex CM19 5BQ. Tel: 0800 801405.

MeReC Bulletin provides reviews of new drugs aimed at GPs covering issues of safety, effectiveness, cost, appropriateness and acceptability. It is available from the Medicines Resource Centre, Hamilton House, 24 Pall Mall, Liverpool L3 6AL.

Netting the Evidence is part of the Cochrane Library that advises on where to find information on the Internet on using evidence in practice. See http://www.nettingtheevidence.org.uk.

NHS Economic Evaluation Database provides critiques of published economic evaluations. It is available from the NHS Centre for Reviews and Dissemination, University of York, York YO1 5DD or on the Internet at http://nhscrd.york.ac.uk/welcome.html.

Organisations

Aggressive Research Intelligence Facility (ARIF)
ARIF is a specialist unit funded by the NHS Executive, West Midlands. The role of the unit is to improve the incorporation

of research findings into population-level healthcare decisions in the NHS by helping healthcare workers access and interpret research evidence, particularly systematic reviews of research. Although ARIF has a regional role, it will attempt to help all callers. The website provides summaries of the research information ARIF has uncovered in response to requests received. The website is at: http://www.bham.ac.uk/arif/.

National Institute for Clinical Excellence (NICE)
NICE provides NHS patients, health professionals and the public in England and Wales with authoritative, robust and reliable guidance on current 'best practice'. This is regularly updated and offers guidance on appraisals of new and existing health technologies, the clinical management of specific conditions and clinical audit. Information about the Institute and its work is available on their website at: www.nice.org.uk.

NHS Centre for Reviews and Dissemination (CRD)
CRD is a sibling organisation of the UK Cochrane Centre, funded by the Department of Health to provide information on the effectiveness and cost-effectiveness of treatments and the delivery and organisation of healthcare. CRD carries out systematic reviews, provides a database of good quality reviews, offers a dissemination and information service and helps to promote research-based practice in the NHS. CRD plays an important role in disseminating the contents of Cochrane reviews to NHS decision makers. It provides an information and enquiry service on reviews and economic evaluations for healthcare professionals, purchasers and providers, NHS managers, information providers, health service researchers and consumer organisations. Its main outputs are: *Effective Healthcare Bulletins*; *Effectiveness Matters*; Database of Abstracts of Reviews of Effectiveness (DARE); NHS Economic Evaluation Database (NHS EED); and the Health Technology Assessment (HTA) Database. NHS Centre for Reviews and Dissemination, University of York, York YO1 5DD. Tel: 01904 433707. Email: revdis@york.ac.uk. The website is at: http://www.york.ac.uk/inst/crd/.

Useful websites include:
- Centre for Evidence-Based Medicine:
  http://cebm.jr2.ox.ac.uk/
- Clinical Governance Research and Development Unit:
  http://www.le.ac.uk/cgrdu
- Cochrane Collaboration Home Page:
  http://hiru.mcmaster.ca/cochrane/default.htm
- EBM Informatics Home Page:
  http://hiru.hirunet.mcmaster.ca/ebm/
- EBM toolbox:
  http://cebm.jr2.ox.ac.uk/
- IDEA Topics List:
  www.ohsu.edu/bicc-informatics/ebm/ebm_topics.htm
- Netting the Evidence:
  http://www.nettingtheevidence.org.uk
- 'NEW' TRIP database: http://www.tripdatabase.com/
- Trawling the Net:
  http://www.shef.ac.uk~scharr/ir/trawling.html
- Ukpractice.net Ltd: http://www.ukpractice.net

There is also a very good email discussion group: evidence-based-health@mailbase.ac.uk.

To join send the following email to mailbase@mailbase.ac.uk. Leave the subject field empty and type the message 'join evidence-based-health Jo Bloggs'. To get the list of discussions, send the email. Website at http://www.mailbase.ac.uk.

Further reading

Baker M, Maskrey N and Kirk S (1997) *Clinical Effectiveness and Primary Care*. Radcliffe Medical Press, Oxford.

Chambers R and Wakley G (2000) *Making Clinical Governance Work for You*. Radcliffe Medical Press, Oxford.

Crombie I (1996) *The Pocket Guide to Critical Appraisal*. BMJ Publishing Group, London.

Greenhalgh T (1997) *How to Read a Paper: the basics of evidence-based medicine.* BMJ Publishing Group, London.

Jones R and Kinmonth AL (eds) (1995) *Critical Reading for Primary Care.* Oxford University Press, Oxford.

The King's Fund (1998) *Turning Evidence into Everyday Practice.* The King's Fund, London.

Kobelt G (1996) *Health Economics: an introduction to economic evaluation.* Office of Health Economics, London.

Lilley R (1999) *Making Sense of Clinical Governance.* Radcliffe Medical Press, Oxford.

Muir Gray JA (1997) *Evidence-Based Healthcare.* Churchill Livingstone, Edinburgh.

Ridsdale L (1995) *Evidence-Based General Practice.* Saunders, London.

Sackett D, Richardson S, Rosenberg W and Haynes RB (1997) *Evidence-Based Medicine.* Churchill Livingstone, Edinburgh.

van Zwanenberg T and Harrison J (eds) (2000) *Clinical Governance in Primary Care.* Radcliffe Medical Press, Oxford.

Wilson T (ed) (1999) *The PCG Development Guide.* Radcliffe Medical Press, Oxford.

Computer language

Internet acronyms:

AFAIK: as far as I know
AKA: also known as
BTW: by the way
FAQ: frequently asked question
FYI: for your information
IM(H)O: in my (humble) opinion
NRN: no response necessary
TIA: thanks in advance
TTFN: ta ta for now
WRT: with respect to.

► REFERENCES

1 NHS Executive (1996) *Promoting Clinical Effectiveness*. NHS Executive, London.

2 Hicks N (1997) Evidence-based health care. *Bandolier*. 4(5): 8.

3 Sackett DL, Rosenberg WM, Gray J, Haynes RB and Richardson WS (1996) Evidence-based medicine: what it is and what it isn't. *BMJ*. **312**: 71–2.

4 Haynes B, Sackett D, Gray JM, Cook D and Guyatt G (1996) Transferring evidence from research into practice: 1. The role of clinical care research evidence in clinical decisions. *Evidence-Based Medicine*. **November/December**: 196–7.

5 Haynes B, Sackett D, Gray JM, Cook D and Guyatt G (1997) Transferring evidence from research into practice: 4. Overcoming barriers to application. *Evidence-Based Medicine*. **May/June**: 68–9.

6 The King's Fund (1997) *Turning Evidence into Everyday Practice*. The King's Fund, London.

7 McColl A, Smith H, White P and Field J (1998) General practitioners' perceptions of the route to evidence-based medicine: a questionnaire survey. *BMJ*. **316**: 361–5.

8 Samuel O (1997) Evidence-based general practice: what is needed right now. *Audit Trends*. **5**: 111–15.

9 Prescott K, Lloyd M, Douglas HR *et al.* (1997) Promoting clinically effective practice: general practitioners' awareness of sources of evidence. *Fam Pract*. **14**: 320–3.

10 Paterson C (1997) Problem setting and problem solving: the role of evidence-based medicine. *J Roy Soc Med*. **90**: 304–6.

11 le Vann T (1998) Are we doing any good? *Monitor.* **4 February**: 19.

12 Kernick D (1997) Why GPs should be wary of evidence-based medicine. *Pulse.* **13 December**: 48–50.

13 Houghton G and Mendes da Costa B (1997) *EBM: a multidisciplinary educational needs assessment in the West Midlands* (unpublished). Evidence-supported Medicine Union, 27 Highfield Road, Edgbaston, Birmingham B15 3DP.

14 NHS Executive West Midlands (1995) *GRIP Kit, 1995.* The GRIP Group, NHS Executive West Midlands.

15 Royal College of General Practitioners (1993) *Portfolio-based Learning in General Practice: a report of a working group on higher professional education.* Occasional Paper 63. RCGP, London.

16 Treasure W (1996) Portfolio-based learning pilot scheme for general practitioner principals in South East Scotland. *Education for General Practice.* 7: 249–54.

17 Burrows P and Millard L (1996) Personal learning in general practice. *Education for General Practice.* 7: 300–5.

18 United Kingdom Central Council for Nursing, Midwifery and Health Visiting (1995) *PREP and You: maintaining your registrations. Standards for education following registration.* UKCC fact sheets. UKCC, London.

19 Millman A, Lee N and Kealy K (1995) The Internet. ABC of Medical Computing series. *BMJ.* **311**: 440–3.

20 *The Cochrane Library.* Update Software Ltd, Summertown Pavilion, Middle Way, Summertown, Oxford OX2 7LG. http://www.cochrane.co.uk.

21 Brenner SH and McKinnin EJ (1989) CINAHL and Medline: a comparison of indexing practices. *Bulletin of the Medical Library Association.* 77: 366–71.

22 Okuma E (1994) Selecting CD-ROM databases for nursing students: a comparison of Medline and the Cumulative Index to Nursing and Allied Health Literature (CINAHL). *Bulletin of the Medical Library Association.* **82**: 25–9.

23 Watson MM and Perrin R (1994) A comparison of CINAHL and Medline CD-ROM in four allied health areas. *Bulletin of the Medical Library Association.* **82**: 214–16.

24 Kiley R (1997) Medical databases on the Internet – part 2. *J Roy Soc Med.* **90**: 679–80.

25 Kiley R (1997) How to get medical information from the Internet. *J Roy Soc Med.* **90**: 488–9.

26 Kiley R (1998) Evidence-based medicine on the Internet. *J Roy Soc Med.* **91**: 74–5.

27 *Oxford Clinical Mentor* is available from Janet Caldwell, Oxford University Press, Great Clarendon Street, Oxford OX2 6DP.

28 Muir Gray JA (1997) *Evidence-Based Healthcare.* Churchill Livingstone, Edinburgh.

29 Kobelt G (1996) *Health Economics: an introduction to economic evaluation.* Office of Health Economics, London.

30 Barton S (ed) (2000) *Clinical Evidence. Issue 4.* BMJ Publishing Group, London.

31 Rowlands J, Morrow T, Lee N and Millman A (1995) Online searching. ABC of Medical Computing series. *BMJ.* **311**: 500–4.

32 Greenhalgh T and Taylor R (1997) How to read a paper: papers that go beyond numbers (qualitative research). *BMJ.* **315**: 740–3.

33 Hoddinott P and Pill R (1997) A review of recently published qualitative research in general practice. More methodological questions than answers? *Family Practice.* **14**(4): 313–19.

34 Blaxter M (1996) Criteria for evaluation of qualitative research. *Medical Sociology News.* **22:** 68–71.

35 Mays N and Pope C (eds) (1996) *Qualitative Research in Health Care.* BMJ Publishing Group, London.

36 Mays N and Pope C (2000) Qualitative research in health care. Assessing quality in qualitative research. *BMJ.* **320:** 50–2.

37 Murphy E, Dingwall R, Greatbatch D, Parker S and Watson P (1998) Qualitative research methods in health technology

assessment: a review of the literature. *Health Technology Assessment.* **2**.

38 Waddell G, McIntosh A, Hutchinson A, Feder G and Lewis M (1999) *Low Back Pain Evidence Review.* Royal College of General Practitioners, London.

39 Black D (1998) The limitations of evidence. *Journal of Royal College of Physicians of London.* **32**: 23–6.

40 Lilley R (1999) *Making Sense of Clinical Governance.* Radcliffe Medical Press, Oxford.

41 Department of Health (1997) *The New NHS: modern, dependable.* The Stationery Office, London.

42 Department of Health (1998) *A First Class Service: quality in the new NHS.* Health Services Circular HSC (98)113. Department of Health, London.

43 Chambers R and Wakley G (2000) *Making Clinical Governance Work for You.* Radcliffe Medical Press, Oxford.

44 Lilley R and Lambden P (2000) *Making Sense of Risk Management.* Radcliffe Medical Press, Oxford.

45 Wakley G, Chambers R and Field S (2000) *Continuing Professional Development in Primary Care: making it happen.* Radcliffe Medical Press, Oxford.

46 Royal College of General Practitioners (2000) *Quality Team Development.* RCGP, London.

47 Dunning M, Abi-Aad G, Gilbert D *et al.* (1999) *Experience, Evidence and Everyday Practice.* King's Fund, London.

48 Taylor M (1995) *Unleashing the Potential: bringing residents to the centre of regeneration.* Joseph Rowntree Foundation, York.

49 Chambers R (2000) *Involving Patients and the Public: how to do it better.* Radcliffe Medical Press, Oxford.

50 Department of Health (1997) *Report of the review of patient-identifiable information.* In: *The Caldicott Committee Report.* Department of Health, London.

51 Donald P (2000) Promoting local ownership of guidelines. *Guidelines in Practice.* **3**: 17.

52 English National Board (1996) *Supervision of Midwives: the English National Board's advice and guidance to LSAs and supervisors of midwives*. ENB, London.

53 United Kingdom Central Council (1998) *Midwives Rules and Code of Practice*. UKCC, London.

54 Mohanna K and Chambers R (2001) *Risk Matters in Healthcare: communicating, explaining and managing risk*. Radcliffe Medical Press, Oxford.

55 NHS Executive (1999) *The NHS Performance Assessment Framework*. Department of Health, London.

56 NHS Executive (1999) *Primary Care Trusts: establishing better services*. NHSE, London.

57 Dewar S (1999) *Clinical Governance Under Construction*. King's Fund, London.

58 James A (2000) Making space for clinical governance. *Impact in Bandolier*. 7(3): 5–6.

► INDEX